Fructose Malabsorption
The Shopping Guide

Debra & Bob Ledford

To order additional books, please contact:

help@fructosemalabsorptionhelp.com
or
Ledford Publishing
P.O. Box 6756
Brookings, OR 97415

Send comments, questions, corrections, or information to:
help@fructosemalabsorptionhelp.com

About this Guide

Whether you are new to FM, and still trying to find something to eat, or have more experience than you care to, this guide will assist in your search for foods which should be safe for an FMer.

Will there be foods in this guide you cannot eat? Probably. Will there be foods you eat, but are not in this guide? Almost certainly. Since we have attempted to compile a list of foods acceptable to as many FMer's as possible, there are certain ingredients you may find acceptable, which have been excluded in this guide, such as corn and chocolate. If you are fortunate enough to tolerate such ingredients, you may add to the list.

With that said, as usual, there are exceptions to the rule. When we were unable to locate any (or very few) acceptable items, but found one with a questionable ingredient, we have included it. For example, we were unable to find ice cream cones other than Goldbaum's, which has cocoa powder, so it was included. Also, being aware that some can tolerate corn, we have included a few cold cereals with corn in the ingredients due to the small selection of acceptable cold cereals available.

The Foods

A large number of the foods in this guide are organic. Most prepared foods in the average grocery store contain unacceptable ingredients for FMer's. Thankfully, more and more grocers are now carrying a selection of organic foods, so you may be able to locate them at your neighborhood grocer. If not, an occasional trip to the nearest organic foods store will be worth the effort. We travel three hours to get to the nearest one to us.

If still unable to locate foods listed, you can request for your local store to begin carrying them, or order them online.

Entries

Every attempt has been made to include information which will help you determine if an item is acceptable to you. Each listing contains:
- Product name, listed by brand
- Internet address, when available
- Ingredients
- Dietary notes as listed on packaging or website, with sugar grams, if any

While we encourage you to carefully read the ingredients as listed, DO NOT rely on these when shopping. Manufacturers regularly change their products and the ingredients can and do change. Always read the package label, even on items you purchase regularly.

Suggestion: Use a pen or highlighter when reading through each listing. If there are questionable ingredients for you, mark it. If you know an item is unacceptable for you, cross it out. Add items you can eat which are not included (and let us know).

Notable

A few of the ingredient lists include terms like "spices" and "natural flavors." We have attempted, when possible, to discover the actual spices and natural flavors, but responses to our queries were usually a form e-mail which did not answer the question asked. Be aware these may or may not be acceptable. We suggest you trial them if needed.

Some of the items contain sugar. Since sugar (sucrose) is a 50/50 fructose/glucose ratio, it is acceptable for FMer's in small amounts. To assist the FMer in determining if they are willing to try an item, we have included the sugar grams for each item.

This symbol indicates the item should be acceptable for the new FMer who is still in the cleansing phase and has not yet started trialing foods, assuming they do not have other dietary intolerances, such as lactose or eggs.

Guide to Dietary Notes

CF - Corn Free
DF - Dairy Free
CSF - Caisson Free
EF - Egg Free
FT - Fair Trade
GF - Gluten Free
MSGF - MSG Free
Non-GMO - Free of genetically modified organisms

PF - Peanut Free
SF - Soy Free
SUN - Sugar Gram Information Unavailable
TNF - Tree Nut Free
WF - Wheat Free
YF - Yeast Free

Cost of Foods

For those of you who are new to organic foods, you may go through a bit of sticker shock. Yes, they are more expensive, though how much more may depend upon where you shop. We see food as a "pay now, or pay later" item. Either pay now for healthy foods, or pay later for medical problems.

To help ease the sticker shock, we had hoped to include manufacturer coupons in this book, but much to our regret, we were unable to arrange this. We did, however, get a few coupon codes to use when ordering online:

Brothers-All-Natural - *BANFM15* - 15% off order, no expiration date
　　　Free shipping anywhere in continental U.S. with $25 order
NuNaturals - *BLG0614* - 15% off order, expires 6/30/2014
　　　Free shipping anywhere in continental U.S. with $35 order,
　　　excluding discounts
Julian Bakery - *1776* - $5 off on-line orders, no expiration date

The savings should not stop here. Take the time and go on many of the company websites to receive coupons. By doing this, I received $48.35 in coupons for items listed in this book. Beware, some stores do not accept on-line printed coupons, so know your store's coupon policy. Also, these coupons usually have an expiration date only two to thirty days out.
Though coupons come and go, some of the sites on which I found coupons are:

Arrowhead Mills
Bisquick
Bob's Red Mill
Glutino
Go Veggie!
Hinode Rice
Jennie O
La Preferida Lundberg
MiraLax
Nature Made
Saputo Cheese USA
Silk
Stonyfield
Valley Fresh

Below is a list of some of the *ingredients we have avoided* in this guide. While these may be okayingredients for someFMer's, others react, so we have tried to avoid them in this book. (Remember, there are exceptions to this rule, so read the listed ingredients carefully.)

- agave
- apple
- artichoke
- asparagus
- aspartame
- avocado
- barley
- beet
- brown rice
- brown sugar
- cabbage
- canola oil
- cellulose
- cherry
- chives
- chocolate
- coconut
- corn syrup
- corn syrup solids
- cucumber
- date
- date sugar
- fructose
- fruit juice sweeteners
- garbanzo beans (chickpeas)
- garlic
- ginger
- grape
- high fructose corn syrup
- honey
- inulin
- invert sugar
- isoglucose
- isomalt
- leek
- lentils
- levulose
- mango
- maltitol
- molasses
- maltose
- maple syrup
- onion
- paprika
- peach
- pear
- peas
- pineapple
- plum
- raisins
- rye
- saccharin
- shallot
- sorbitol
- soy
- Splenda
- sucralose
- sucrose syrup
- tomato (paste, sauce, etc)
- vegetable oil
- watermelon
- wheat
- xylitol

Shopping List

This is a generic shopping list. If you have other food intolerances, you will need to cross those foods off the list. Certainly, you should add to the list if your tolerance levels allow. As always, read package ingredients.

Dairy
- butter[1]
- cheese[2]
- cottage cheese
- cream
- milk
- sour cream

Proteins (not processed/breaded)
- almonds
- eggs
- hazelnuts
- meat - unprocessed (any kind - chicken, pork, beef, buffalo, venison, fish, shellfish, etc.)
- peanuts
- seeds

Grains
- millet
- oats
- polenta
- quinoa
- rice

Drinks
- coffee
- dry wine
- rum
- tea[3]
- vodka

Misc.
- olive oil
- pumpkin seeds

Fruit*
- bananas
- blueberries
- grapefruit
- kiwi
- lemons
- limes
- oranges
- strawberries

Vegetables*
- alfalfa
- bean sprouts
- broccoli
- butternut squash
- carrots*
- celery
- green bell pepper
- olives
- potatoes
- pumpkin
- red chili
- romaine lettuce
- snow peas*
- spinach, baby (remove stem)
- tomatoes*
- yams*
- zucchini

Herbs
- basil
- coriander
- oregano
- parsley
- rosemary

---

* limit quantity
1 not margarine
2 Pre-shredded/grated usually contains cellulose as an anti-clumping agent, which can be problematic - read ingredients on any cheese
3 be sure to read ingredients - we highly recommend *Good Earth Sweet and Spicy* - there is no sweetener of any kind added but tastes like there is

Baking Needs

Bob's Red Mill Active Dry Yeast

www.bobsredmill.com
Ingredients: sodium bicarbonate

Notes: GF Manufactured in a facility that also uses tree nuts and soy.

Bob's Red Mill Baking Soda

www.bobsredmill.com
Ingredients: active dry yeast

Notes: GF Manufactured in a facility that also uses tree nuts and soy.

Bob's Red Mill Double Acting Baking Powder
www.bobsredmill.com
Ingredients: sodium acid pyrophosphate, sodium bicarbonate, corn starch, monocalcium phosphate

Notes: GF Manufactured in a facility that also uses tree nuts and soy.

Bob's Red Mill Guar Gum
www.bobsredmill.com
Ingredients: guar gum
Notes: GF Manufactured in a facility that also uses tree nuts and soy. Guar gum is a flour-like substance made from an East Indian seed. Use small amounts as a thickener, binder, and volume enhancer. Instructions for use on package.

Bob's Red Mill Pie Crust
www.bobsredmill.com
Ingredients: rice flour, potato starch, tapioca flour, sugar, rice bran, sea salt, xanthan gum

Notes: GF, WF, DF, 2g Sugar Manufactured in a facility that also uses tree nuts and soy.

Bob's Red Mill Xanthan Gum
www.bobsredmill.com
Ingredients: xanthan gum
Notes: GF, Manufactured in a facility that also uses tree nuts and soy. Xanthan Gum is used to add volume and viscosity to bread and other gluten-free baked goods. It is made from a tiny microorganism called Xanthomonas campestris and is a natural carbohydrate.

Bragg Nutritional Yeast Seasoning

www.bragg.com
Ingredients: inactive dry yeast, niacin (B3), pyridoxine HCI (B6), riboflavin (B2), thiamin HCI (B1), folic acid, vitamin B12

Notes: GF, Non-GMO, Vegan, Kosher

Baking Needs - Continued

Let's Do...Organic Tapioca Starch
www.edwardandsons.com

Ingredients: organic tapioca starch
,

Notes: GF, Non-GMO, Vegan Great alternative to corn starch

Manischewitz Potato Starch

www.manischewitz.com

Ingredients: potato starch

Notes:

Natural Desserts Unflavored Jel Dessert
www.

Ingredients: vegetable gum, adipic acid, tapioca dextrin, calcium phosphate, potassium citrate

Notes: GF, Vegan

Pomona's Universal Pectin
www.pomonapectin.com

Ingredients: 1 packet low methoxyl citrus pectin, 1 packet monocalcium phosphate

Notes: GF, Non-GMO, Vegan, Kosher This can make low sugar or even no sweetener jelly. It can also be used for aspic, jello, sorbet, yogurt, pie, milk, and candy.

Bread & Baked

Against the Grain Baggetts—Original and Rosemary
www.againstthegraingourmet.com
Ingredients: tapioca starch, milk, eggs, mozzarella cheese, non-GMO canola oil, salt, (rosemary)

Notes: GF

Against The Grain Rolls—Original and Rosemary
www.againstthegraingourmet.com
Ingredients: tapioca starch, milk, eggs, mozzarella cheese, non-GMO canola oil, salt, (rosemary)

Notes: GF

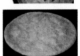

Against The Grain Pizza Shell
www.againstthegraingourmet.com
Ingredients: tapioca starch, milk, eggs, non-GMO canola oil, mozzarella cheese, cheddar cheese , parmesan cheese

Notes: GF

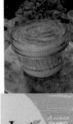

Compelled Bakery Luscious Lemon Cupcake
www.compelledbakery.com
Ingredients: Base - organic eggs, organic evaporated cane juice, gluten-free potato starch, lemon juice **Frosting -** cream cheese, vegan margarine, powdered sugar, lemon juice, vanilla

Notes: GF, SUN

Ian's Gluten Free Panko Original
www.iansnaturalfoods.com
Ingredients: rice flour, xanthan gum, salt, leavening (sodium bicarbonate, gluconolactone), canola oil, sugar, yeast, ascorbic acid

Notes: GF, LF, CSF, EF, TNF Made in a facility that manufactures products containing soy.

Whole Foods Almond Scones
www.wholefoodsmarket.com
Ingredients: rice flour, RBGH free butter (cream), heavy cream, evaporated cane juice, cage free eggs, tapioca starch, potato starch, almond meal (almonds), almonds, baking powder (sodium acid pyrophosphate, sodium bicarbonate, cornstarch, monocalcium phosphate), natural almond flavor, xanthan gum, salt
Notes: GF, SUN

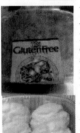

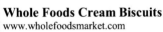

Whole Foods Cream Biscuits
www.wholefoodsmarket.com
Ingredients: heavy cream, rice flour, potato starch, tapioca starch, baking powder (sodium acid pyrophosphate, sodium bicarbonate, cornstarch, monocalcium phosphate), evaporated cane juice, salt, xanthan gum
Notes: GF, SUN

Bread & Baked- Continued

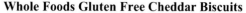

Whole Foods Gluten Free Cheddar Biscuits

Ingredients: heavy cream, rice flour, buttermilk (cultured fat-free milk, salt, vitamin a palmitate, vitamin D3) potato starch, tapioca starch, cheddar cheese (pasteurized cow's milk, cheese culture, salt, enzymes, annatto) baking powder (sodium acid pyrophosphate, bicarbonate soda, cornstarch, monocalcium phosphate), evaporated cane juice, parmesan cheese (pasteurized part-skim milk, cheese culture, salt, enzymes), salt, xanthan gum, chives

Notes: GF, SUN

Whole Foods Gluten Free Sandwich Bread

www.wholefoodsmarket.com

Ingredients: nonfat milk, rice flour, tapioca starch, cage free eggs, evaporated cane juice, canola oil, yeast salt, xanthan gum, lemon juice

Notes: GF, SUN

Whole Foods Gluten Stuffing Cubes

www.wholefoodsmarket.com

Ingredients: nonfat milk, rice flour, tapioca starch, cage free eggs, evaporated cane juice, canola oil, yeast salt, xanthan gum, lemon juice

Notes: GF, SUN

Bread Mixes

123 Gluten Free - Aaron's Favorite Rolls
www.shop123glutenfree.com
Ingredients: rice flour, tapioca flour, Indian rice grass flour (perennial bunch grass, achnatherum hymenoides), sugar, salt, xanthan gum, gluten-free yeast packet

Notes: GF, WF, DF, CSF, PF, TNF, CF, EF, SF, Non-GMO, 2g Sugar

123 Gluten Free - Meredith's Marvelous Muffin/ Quickbread
www.shop123glutenfree.com
Ingredients: rice flour, sugar, tapioca flour, potato starch, baking soda, salt, aluminum-free corn-free baking powder (sodium acid pyrophosphate, baking soda, potato starch, monocalcium phosphate), spices, xanthan gum
Notes: GF, WF, CSF, DF, PF, TNF, CF, EF, SF, Non-GMO, 6g Sugar

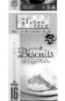

123 Gluten Free - Southern Glory Biscuits
www.shop123glutenfree.com
Ingredients: rice flour, tapioca flour, potato starch, corn starch, aluminum-free baking powder (sodium acid pyrophosphate, baking soda, corn starch, monocalcium phosphate), xanthan gum, salt

Notes: GF, WF, DF, CSF, PF, TNF, EF, SF, Non-GMO, 3g Sugar

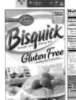

Bisquick Gluten Free Pancake and BakingMix
www.bettycrocker.com
Ingredients: rice flour, sugar, levening (baking soda, sodium aluminum phospahate)

Notes: GF, WF, 3g Sugar May contain soy ingredients.

Bob's Red Mill Biscuit and Baking Mix
www.bobsredmill.com
Ingredients: stone ground white rice flour, garbanzo bean flour, baking powder (sodium acid pyrophosphate, sodium bicarbonate, corn starch, monocalcium phosphate), xanthan gum, sea salt (magnesium carbonate as flowing agent)
Notes: GF, WF, DF Manufactured in a facility that also uses tree nuts and soy.

Chēbē
www.chebe.com
Ingredients: stone ground white rice flour, garbanzo bean flour, baking powder (sodium manioc (tapioca) flour, modified manioc starch, iodine-free sea salt, cream of tartar, sodium bicarbonate, rosemary, basil
Notes: GF, WF, CF, SF,YF, PF, TNF, CSF, LF, Non-GMO, Kosher Made on equipment shared with eggs

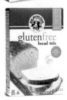

King Arthur Flour Gluten Free Bread Mix
www.kingarthurflour.com
Ingredients: bread mix specialty blend (rice flour, tapioca starch), tapioca starch, **sugar**, emulsifier (rice starch, polyglycerol esters of fatty acids, mono– and diglycerides of fatty acids), salt, xanthan gum, calcium carbonate, niacinamide (a b vitamin), reduced iron, thiamin hydrochloride (vitamin b1), riboflavin (vitamin b2), dry yeast: yeast, sorbotan monostearate, ascorbic acid
Notes: GF, WF, 2g Sugar

Broth/Gravy/Sauces

Pacific Organic Turkey Gravy

www.pacificfoods.com

Ingredients: organic turkey broth (water, organic turkey), roux (organic turkey flour, organic turkey fat), organic crème fraiche (cultured organic cream-milk), organic roasted turkey, sea salt, organic rosemary extract

Notes:

Marukan Ponzu Natural Citrus Marinade

www.marukan-usa.com

Ingredients: concentrated lemon juice, vinegar, citrus (sudachi) juice, citric acid, salt, natural flavor

Notes: GF, Non-GMO

Savory Choice Beef Broth

www.savorychoice.com

Ingredients: beef stock, natural flavor, salt, beef fat, sugar, maltodextrin, yeast extract, xanthan gum

Notes: GF, MSGF, < 1g Sugar

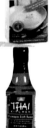

Savory Choice Chicken Broth

www.savorychoice.com

Ingredients: chicken stock, natural flavor, salt, chicken fat, sugar, maltodextrin, yeast extract, xanthan gum

Notes: GF, MSGF, < 1g Sugar

Thai Kitchen Premium Fish Sauce

www.thaikitchen.com

Ingredients: anchovy extract, salt, unrefined cane sugar

Notes: GF, DF, may contain peanuts, < 1 g sugar

Cake/Frosting Mixes

123 Gluten Free - Delightfully Gratifying Bundt Poundcake
www.shop123glutenfree.com
Ingredients: sugar, rice flour, potato starch, tapioca flour, aluminum-free corn-free baking powder (sodium acid pyrophosphate, baking soda, potato starch, monocalcium phosphate), natural flavor, xanthan gum
Notes: GF, WF, DF, CSF, PF, CF, TNF, EF, SF, Non-GMO, 31g Sugar

123 Gluten Free - Yummy Yellow Cake Mix
www.shop123glutenfree.com
Ingredients: rice flour, potato starch, tapioca starch, aluminum-free corn-free baking powder (sodium acid pyrophosphate, baking soda, potato starch, monocalcium phosphate), natural flavor, xanthan gum, salt
Notes: GF, WF, DF, CSF, PF, CF, TNF, EF, SF, Non-GMO, < 1g Sugar (add your own)

Bob's Red Mill Vanilla Cake Mix
www.bobsredmill.com
Ingredients: sugar, potato starch, tapioca flour, whole grain sorghum flour, baking powder (monocalcium phosphate, bicarbonate of soda, cornstarch), sea salt (magnesium phosphate as a flowing agent), xanthan gum, natural vanilla powder (sugar, corn starch, vanilla extract)
Notes: GF, WF, DF, 16g Sugar Manufactured in a facility that also uses tree nuts and soy.

Dawd & Rogers Gluten Free Dark Vanilla Cake Mix
www.dowdandrogers.com
Ingredients: organic evaporated cane juice, gourmet flour blend (fine white rice flour, Italian chestnut flour, tapioca flour), cultured buttermilk, pure vanilla powder, aluminum-free baking powder, salt, xanthan gum, baking soda
Notes: GF, WF, 24g Sugar

Dawd & Rogers Gluten Free Golden Lemon Cake Mix
www.dowdandrogers.com
Ingredients: organic evaporated cane juice, gourmet flour blend (fine white rice flour, Italian chestnut flour, tapioca flour), cultured buttermilk, natural lemon flavor powder, aluminum-free baking powder, salt, xanthan gum, baking soda
Notes: GF, WF, 24g Sugar

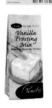

Glutino Gluten Free Pantry Old Fashioned Yellow Cake Mix
www.glutino.com
Ingredients: white rice flour, sugar, potato starch, sodium bicarbonate, xanthan gum, salt, sodium acid pyrophosphate, monocalcium phosphate

Notes: GF, Non-GMO, 14g Sugar

Pamela's Vanilla Frosting Mix
www.pamalasproducts.com
Ingredients: organic powdered sugar (contains 3% corn starch), gluten free natural vanilla powder, sea salt

Notes: GF, WF, 22g Sugar

Candy/Gum

Remember, regardless of the ingredients, this is still candy, which means sugar. Even used medicinally, as glucose to counter fructose, it must be limited. If you should choose to indulge, be sure to keep the servings very small and infrequent. Also, double-check the ingredients. We include this section to assist those who are searching for *any* possibilities for treats, not because they are a sure-thing for all FMer's.

Altoids Curiously Strong Mints - Liquorice
www.altoids.com
Ingredients: sugar, natural flavors, gum Arabic, gelatin

Notes: 2g Sugar Check ingredients on other flavors. When in the store, the tins has unacceptable ingredients, but a recent check of the website showed they were essentially the same as liquorice.

Bissinger's Raspberry Yumberry Gummy Pandas
www.bissingers.com
Ingredients: organic tapioca syrup, organic cane sugar, gelatin, dried raspberry powder, citric acid, lactic acid, natural flavor, ascorbic acid, organic yumberry powder, color (organic black carrot juice concentrate), organic sunflower oil, carnauba wax
Notes: GF, 19g Sugar Packed in a facility that also uses milk, soy, peanuts, tree nuts, wheat and eggs.

Glee Gum - Peppermint
www.gleegum.com
Ingredients: cane sugar, glucose, gum base (contains natural chicle), brown rice syrup, natural peppermint flavor, gum Arabic, resinous glaze, beeswax, carnauba wax, chlorophyll
Notes: Non-GMO, FT, Kosher, 2g Sugar Ingredients vary by flavor. No artificial flavors or colors.

Gummy Zone Gummy Candy Hot Dogs

Ingredients: glucose syrup, sugar, water, gelatin, citric acid, artificial flavors, carnauba wax, artificial colors (red 40, yellow 5, yellow 6, blue 1, titanium dioxide)

Notes: 22g Sugar

Smarties
www.smarties.com
Ingredients: dextrose, citric acid, calcium stearate, natural and artificial flavors, colors (red 40 lake, yellow 5 lake, yellow 6 lake, blue 2 lake
Notes: GF, WF, SF, EF, PF, TNF, Vegan, 6g Sugar See re-bagger info on their allergen info page. Can allow small amounts of fructose to be absorbed. Does not work with fructans.

Extreme Sour Smarties
www.smarties.com
Ingredients: dextrose, citric acid, calcium stearate, natural and artificial flavors, colors (red 40 lake, yellow 5 lake, yellow 6 lake, blue 2 lake
Notes: GF, WF, SF, EF, PF, TNF, Vegan, 6g Sugar
See re-bagger info on their allergen info page.

Candy/Gum - Continued

Yummy Earth - Organic Gummy Bears

www.yummyearth.com

Ingredients: organic rice syrup, organic cane sugar, gelatin, organic aronia juice, organic black currant juice, natural flavor, citric acid, ascorbic acid, carnuba wax, organic sunflower oil

Notes: EG, PF, TNF, WF, SF, DF, MSGF, 15g Sugar 100% natural flavors & colors,. Though it contains juice, I am able to eat a few without problems.

Yummy Earth - Organic Lollypops

www.yummyearth.com

Ingredients: organic evaporated cane juice, organic tapioca syrum/organic rice syrup, citric acid (from beet sugar), natural flavors, may contain organic black carrows, organic black currants, organic pumpkin, organic apple, organic carrot, organic alfalfa

Notes: EG, PF, TNF, WF, SF, MSGF, Kosher, 17g Sugar, 100% natural flavors & colors,. Though it contains juice, I am able to eat one without problems.

Yummy Earth - Sour Beans

www.yummyearth.com

Ingredients: natural sugar, glucose syrup (from tapioca, corn, or rice) modified food starch (from tapioca, corn, or rice), fumaric acid (for sour), ascorbic acid (for vitamin C), natural flavors, acacia gum, purple carrot juice, beta carotene.

Notes: EG, PF, TNF, WF, SF, MSGF, 15g Sugar, 100% natural flavors & colors,. Though it contains juice, I am able to eat a few without problems.

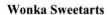

Wonka Pixy Stix

www.wonka.com

Ingredients: dextrose, citric acid, less than 2% of artificial flavors, red 40 lake, yellow 5 lake, yellow 6 lake, blue 2 lake, blue 1 lake

Notes: 15g Sugar

Wonka Sweetarts

www.wonka.com

Ingredients: dextrose, maltodextrin, malic acid,, less than 2% of calcium sterate, artificial flavors, red 40 lake, yellow 5 lake, yellow 6 lake, blue 2 lake, blue 1 lake

Notes: 10.8g Sugar

Canned Meats

This is just a sampling of possible canned meats, many of which come in different types (such as dark chicken, or packed in water). Many FMer's ask what FM friendly foods to put in emergency food supplies; these are great for protein.

Brunswick Kippered Seafood Snacks

www.brunswick.ca

Ingredients: herring fillets, water, salt, natural smoke flavoring sodium hexametaphosphate

Notes:

Brunswick Sardines in Olive Oil

www.brunswick.ca

Ingredients: sardines (fish), olive oil

Notes:

John West Kipper Fillets in Sunflower Oil

www.john-west.co.uk

Ingredients: kipper filets, sunflower oil, salt

Notes:

Pacific Pearl Tiny Shrimp

Ingredients: shrimp, water, salt, sugar, citric acid, sodium bisulfite as a preservative

Notes: 1g sugar

Pacific Pearl Smoked Clams

Ingredients: smoked baby clams, cottonseed oil, salt

Notes:

Spam Classic

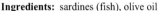

www.spam.com

Ingredients: ham, pork, sugar, salt, water, potato starch, sodium nitrate

Notes: <1g Sugar

Canned Meats - Continued

Starkist Solid White Albacore Tuna

www.starkist.com

Ingredients: tuna, water, vegetable broth, salt, pyrophosphate

Notes:

Swanson Premium Chunk Chicken Breast

www.swansonchicken.com

Ingredients: cooked chicken breast meat, water, contains less than 2% of the following: modified food starch, salt, sodium phosphates

Notes:

Tyson Premium Chunk White Chicken

www.tyson.com

Ingredients: chunk white chicken, water, contain 2%or less of : salt, modified food starch, sodium phosphates, chicken broth, flavorings

Notes:

Valley Fresh 100% Natural Chicken in Water

www.valleyfresh.com

Ingredients: chicken, water, salt

Notes:

Canned Vegetables

This is just a sampling of possible canned veggies, many of which come in different types. Many FMer's ask what FM friendly foods to put in emergency food supplies; these may not be the best cold, but they work.

Farmers Market Organic Butternut Squash
www.farmersmarketfoods.com
Ingredients: certified organic butternut squash

Notes: 4g Sugar

Farmers Market Organic Pumpkin
www.farmersmarketfoods.com
Ingredients: certified organic pumpkin

Notes: 14g Sugar

Ortega Diced Green Chilies
www.ortega.com
Ingredients: fire roasted green chilies (green chilies, water, salt, citric acid, calcium chloride)

Notes: <1g Sugar

Pacific Jellied Organic Cranberry Sauce
www.pacificfoods.com
Ingredients: organic cranberries, organic cane sugar, water

Notes: 26g Sugar

Pacific Whole Organic Cranberry Sauce
www.pacificfoods.com
Ingredients: organic cranberries, organic cane sugar, water

Notes: 29g Sugar

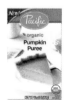

Pacific Organic Pumpkin Puree
www.pacificfoods.com
Ingredients: organic pumpkin

Notes: 4g Sugar

Canned Vegetables - Continued

Reese Hearts of Palm

www.reesespeciality.com

Ingredients: hearts of palm, water, salt, citric acid, ascorbic acid (as anti-oxidant)

Notes: 1g Sugar

Sun Luck Bamboo Shoots

Ingredients: bamboo shoots, water

Notes:

Sun Luck Water Chestnuts

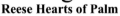

Ingredients: water chestnuts, water

Notes: 1g Sugar

Cereal, Cold

Arrowhead Mills - Puffed Millet

www.arrowheadmills.com
Ingredients: puffed whole grain millet

Notes:

Health Valley Rice Crunch Ums
www.healthvalley.com
Ingredients: milled rice, corn bran, evaporated cane juice, salt, natural vitamin e (added to preserve freshness)

Notes: 2g Sugar Corn - while this cereal does contain corn bran, for some reason I can tolerate it, and I am very sensitive to corn.

Kellogg's Rice Krispies

www.ricekrispies.com
Ingredients: rice, sugar, contains 2 % or less of salt, malt flavor, BHT added to packaging for freshness

Notes: 4g Sugar

Living Intentions Superfood Cereal Hemp & Greens

www.livesuperfoods.com
Ingredients: organic buckwheat sprouts, organic coconut, organic coconut palm sugar, organic banana, organic sultanas, organic sunflower sprouts, raw brown rice bran and germ (grain free), organic sesame seed, green protein superfood blend (organic hemp protein, organic spinach powder, spirulina, chlorella, organic alfalfa leaf, organic dandelion leaf), organic vanilla extract, Himalayan crystal salt
Notes: GF, Vegan, 13g Sugar Processed in a facility that uses tree nuts and peanuts

Nature's Path Envirokids Amazon Frosted Flakes

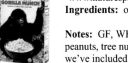

www.naturespath.com
Ingredients: organic corn meal, organic evaporated cane juice, sea salt,

Notes: GF, WF, Non-GMO, 6g Sugar Produced in a facility that uses peanuts, tree nuts, & soy. While this cereal obviously contains corn, we've included it as an option for those who can tolerate corn.

Natures Path Envirokids Gorilla Munch
www.naturespath.com
Ingredients: organic corn meal, organic evaporated cane juice, sea salt

Notes: GF, WF, Non-GMO, 8g Sugar Produced in a facility that uses peanuts, tree nuts, & soy. While this cereal obviously contains corn, we've included it as an option for those who can tolerate corn.

Natures Path Millet Puffs

www.naturespath.com
Ingredients: organic millet

Notes: Non-GMO This product is produced in a plant that contains wheat.

Cereal, Cold - Continued

Natures Path Qi'a Superfood Chia, Buckwheat, & Hemp Cereal Cranberry Vanilla

www.naturespath.com

Ingredients: chia seeds, buckwheat groats, hemp seeds, cranberries (coated with sunflower oil), almonds, natural vanilla flavor

Notes: Non-GMO, 3g Sugar, Organic Contains tree nuts. Produced in a facility that uses soy, peanuts, and dairy

Simple Truth Organic Toasted Oats

www.simpletruth.com

Ingredients: organic whole grain oats (includes the oat bran), organic rice flour, organic sugar, salt, calcium carbonate, mixed tocopherols (vitamin E) added to preserve freshness - vitamins & minerals: ferric orthophosphate, sodium ascorbate, niacinamide, vitamin A acetate, zinc oxide, folic acid, cholecalciferol, thiamine mononitrate, pyridoxine hydrochloride

Note: 1g Sugar May contain wheat, soy, peanuts, almonds

Cereal, Hot

Oatmeal info: Oats are a gluten-free food. However, the problem comes with cross-contamination in the fields. When a bit of wheat grows in with the oats, it may remain in the processing, thus can be problematic. Gluten-free oats assure no cross contamination. We have included both gluten-free and regular oatmeal, since not all FMer's are as sensitive as some.

Annie Chun's Rice Express White Sticky Rice
www.anniechun.com
Ingredients: purified water, sticky white rice, gluconolactone

Notes: GF
Gluconolactone is a natural, non-dairy, gluten-free ingredient derived from corn.)

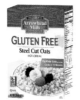

Arrowhead Mills Gluten Free Steel Cut Oats
www.arrowheadmills.com
Ingredients: steel cut oats

Notes: GF, 1g Sugar

Arrowhead Mills Oat Flakes
www.arrowheadmills.com
Ingredients: organic whole grain rolled oats

Notes: <1g Sugar

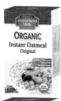

Arrowhead Mills Old Fashioned Oatmeal
www.arrowheadmills.com
Ingredients: organic whole grain rolled oats

Notes: <1g Sugar

Arrowhead Mills Organic Instant Oatmeal
www.arrowheadmills.com
Ingredients: Organic Instant Oatmeal

Notes: <1g Sugar

Arrowhead Mills Organic Oatmeal with Flax
www.arrowheadmills.com
Ingredients: organic instant rolled oats, organic cane sugar, organic golden flax seed, sea salt

Note: 4g Sugar

Cereal, Hot - Continued

Bob's Red Mill Creamy Buckwheat

www.bobsredmill.com
Ingredients: whole grain buckwheat

Notes: Organic, GF, WF
Manufactured in a facility that also uses soy, wheat, and milk.

Bakery on Main Strawberry Shortcake Flavored Instant Oatmeal
www.bakeryonmain.com
Ingredients: certified gluten free oats, evaporated cane juice, freeze dried strawberry, chia seeds, flax meal, quinoa, amaranth, natural flavors, sea salt
Notes: GF, WF, Non GMO, DF, CF, 10g Sugar (Made in a facility that processes tree nuts and peanuts)

Bakery on Main Traditional Flavor Instant Oatmeal
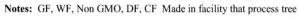
www.bakeryonmain.com
Ingredients: certified gluten free oats, chia seeds, flax meal, quinoa, amaranth

Notes: GF, WF, Non GMO, DF, CF Made in facility that process tree

Bob's Red Mill Millet Grits
www.bobsredmill.com
Ingredients: whole grain millet

Notes: GF
Manufactured in a facility that also uses soy, wheat, and milk.

Country Choice Organic Instant Hot Oatmeal w/Flax
www.countrychoiceorganic.com
Ingredients: organic whole rolled oats, organic milled flaxseed

Notes: Non-GMO, 1g Sugar

Glutenfreeda Instant Oatmeal

www.glutenfreedafoods.com
Ingredients: certified gluten-free oats

Notes: GF, WF, 1g Sugar

Gretchen's Grains Organic Fully Cooked Quinoa—Frozen
www.gretchensgrains.com
Ingredients: quinoa

Notes: 1g Sugar

Cereal, Hot - Continued

Hinode Heat & Serve Jasmine Rice (or White)
www.hinode.us
Ingredients: rice

Notes: GF

Hinode 2 Microwave Cups Jasmine Rice (or White)
www.hinode.us
Ingredients: rice

Notes: GF

Minsley Organic Cooked Quinoa
www.minsley.com
Ingredients: water, organic quinoa, sea salt, glucono delta lactone*

Notes: GF *USDA approved acidifier as an organic ingredient

Minsley Organic Cooked Steelcut Oatmeal
www.minsley.com
Ingredients: organic steelcut oats, water

Notes: 1g Sugar

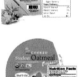

Minsley Cooked White Rice Organic
www.minsley.com
Ingredients: organic white rice, water, glucono delta lactone

Notes: *USDA approved acidifier as an organic ingredient

Natures Path Organic Hot Oatmeal - Original
Www.naturespath.com
Ingredients: organic rolled oats, sea salt

Notes: Non-GMO, 1g Sugar Produced in a facility that uses wheat, tree nuts, and soy.

Roza Thai Jasmine Rice
www.rozafood.com
Ingredients: steamed jasmine rice

Notes:

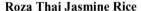

Cereal, Hot - Continued

Thai Kitchen Jasmine Rice
www.thaikitchen.com
Ingredients: jasmine rice (pre-cooked)

Notes: GF, DF, Vegan

Umpqua Oats Jackpot Oatmeal
www.umpquaoats.com
Ingredients: whole rolled oat groats, cane sugar, pecans, freeze-dried raspberries, dried sweetened strawberries (strawberries, sugar), freeze-dried blackberries, sea salt

Notes: 16g Sugar

Umpqua Oats Kick Start Oatmeal
www.umpquaoats.com
Ingredients: whole rolled oat groats, cane sugar, dried sweetened cranberries (cranberries, sugar), brown flax seeds, sunflower seeds, almonds, walnuts, freeze dried wild blueberries, cinnamon, sea salt

Notes: 20g Sugar

Cheese/Cheese Products

Go Veggie American Flavor Slices (or Blocks)
www.goveggiefood.com

Ingredients: organic rice base (filtered water, organic rice flour), **casein** (milk protein), rice bran oil, calcium & sodium phosphate, contains 2% or less of sea salt, rice starch, natural flavors, lactic acid (not-dairy), carageenen, yeast extract (inactive), apocarotinol (color), vitamin A palmitate, riboflavin

Notes: LF, GF, SF, Vegetarian

Go Veggie! also comes in Dairy Free

Go Veggie Cheddar Flavor Slices (or Blocks)
www.goveggiefood.com

Ingredients: organic rice base (filtered water, organic rice flour), **casein** (milk protein), rice bran oil, calcium & sodium phosphate, contains 2% or less of sea salt, rice starch, natural flavors, lactic acid (not-dairy), carageenen, yeast extract (inactive), apocarotinol (color), betacarotine, vitamin A palmitate, riboflavin

Notes: LF, GF, SF, Vegetarian

Go Veggie! also comes in Dairy Free

Go Veggie Mozzarella Flavor Slices (or Blocks)
www.goveggiefood.com

Ingredients: organic rice base (filtered water, organic rice flour), **casein** (milk protein), rice bran oil, calcium & sodium phosphate, contains 2% or less of sea salt, rice starch, natural flavors, lactic acid (not-dairy), carageenen, yeast extract (inactive), vitamin A palmitate, riboflavin

Notes: LF, GF, SF, Vegetarian

Go Veggie! also comes in Dairy Free

Go Veggie Pepper Jack Flavor Slices (or Blocks)
www.goveggiefood.com

Ingredients: organic rice base (filtered water, organic rice flour), **casein** (milk protein), rice bran oil, calcium & sodium phosphate, contains 2% or less of sea salt, rice starch, natural flavors, peppers, (jalapeno, red bell, green bell), lactic acid (not-dairy), carageenen, yeast extract (inactive), vitamin A palmitate, riboflavin

Notes: LF, GF, SF, Vegetarian

Go Veggie! also comes in Dairy Free

Go Veggie Swiss Flavor Slices (or Blocks)
www.goveggiefood.com

Ingredients: organic rice base (filtered water, organic rice flour), **casein** (milk protein), rice bran oil, calcium & sodium phosphate, contains 2% or less of sea salt, rice starch, organic cane sugar, natural flavors, lactic acid (not-dairy), carageenen, yeast extract (inactive), vitamin A palmitate, riboflavin

Notes: LF, GF, SF, Vegetarian

Go Veggie! also comes in Dairy Free

Kaukauna Sharp Cheddar Spreadable Cheese
www.kaukaucheese.com

Ingredients: cheddar cheese (aged over 180 days), pasteurized milk, cheese culture, salt, enzyme, water, reduced lactose whey, cream, sorbic acid (to protect flavor), xanthan gum, lactic acid, salt, apo-carotenol (color)

Notes: 3g Sugar Comes in many flavors—check ingredients.

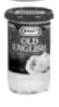

Kraft Old English Cheese Spread

Ingredients: cheddar cheese, (milk, cheese culture, salt, enzymes), water, sodium phosphate, salt, lactic acid, apocarotenal (color)

Notes: This is the only flavor I found that is acceptable.

Cheese/Cheese Products-Continued

Organic Valley Cream Cheese

www.organicvalley.coop
Ingredients: organic pasteurized milk and cream, cheese culture, salt, organic locust bean gum

Notes: kosher, <1g Sugar

Organic Valley Neufchatel Cheese

www.organicvalley.coop
Ingredients: organic pasteurized milk and cream, cheese culture, salt, organic locust bean gum

Notes: kosher, 1g Sugar

Philidelphia Cream Cheese

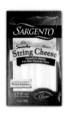

www.kraftbrands.com
Ingredients: pasteurized milk and cream, whey protein concentrate, salt, carob bean gum, cheese culture

Notes: <1g Sugar

Sargento String Cheese

www.sargento.com
Ingredients: pasteurized milk, cheese culture, enzyme, natamycin (mold inhibitor)

Notes:

Chips & Such

Boulder Canyon Totally Natural Kettle Cooked Potato Chips
www.bouldercanyonfoods.com
Ingredients: potatoes, sunflower/safflower oil, salt

Notes: GF, Non-GMO, comes in a totally compostable bag.

CheeCha Original Potato Puffs

www.cheecha.ca
Ingredients: potato flour, potato starch, salt

Notes: GF, DF, TNF, MSGF, Non-GMO

Goldbaums Pop Potato Original
www.goldbaums.com
Ingredients: natural potato ingredients (potato flakes, potato starch), sunflower oil, rice flour, salt

Notes: GF, WF, MSGF, 1g Sugar

Kettle Potato Chips Sea Salt
www.kettlebrand.com
Ingredients: potatoes, vegetable oil (safflower and/or sunflower oil), sea salt

Notes: Non-GMO

Kettle Potato Chips Unsalted
www.kettlebrand.com
Ingredients: potatoes, vegetable oil (safflower and/or sunflower oil)

Notes: Non-GMO

Pik-Nik Original Shoestring Potatoes
www.piknik.com
Ingredients: potato, pure vegetable oil, sea salt

Notes: 1g Sugar

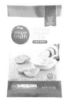

Simple Truth Natural Popped Chips Sea Salt
www.simpletruth.com
Ingredients: potato ingredients (potato flakes, potato starch), sunflower oil, safflower oil and/or canola oil, rice flour, sea salt

Notes: 2g Sugar

Chips & Such - Continued

Simply 7 Quinoa Chips
www.simply7snacks.com
Ingredients: quinoa flour, potato starch, corn starch, expeller pressed safflower oil, corn flour, sugar, sea salt

Notes: GF, Non-GMO, Vegan, Kosher, < 1g Sugar

Wellaby's Cheese Ups Parmesan Cheese
www.wellabys.com
Ingredients: potato starch, edam cheese (cultured milk, salt, enzymes), parmesan cheese (cultured milk, salt, enzymes), egg yolks, yeast extract, milk proteins, salt, natural flavoring

Notes: GF, WF, Non-GMO, MSGF

Wellaby's Cheese Ups Smokehouse
www.wellabys.com
Ingredients: potato starch, edam cheese (cultured milk, salt, enzymes), parmesan cheese (cultured milk, salt, enzymes), egg yolks, yeast extract, milk proteins, salt, natural flavoring

Notes: GF, WF, Non-GMO, MSGF

Condiments

Annie's Organic Dijon Mustard
www.annies.com
Ingredients: distilled white vinegar, mustard seed, sea salt, clove

Notes: Non-GMO, GF

Best Foods Canola Mayonaise
www.bestfoods.com
Ingredients: water, canola oil, modified food starch (corn, potato), eggs, sugar, vinegar, salt, lemon juice, sorbic acid, calcium disodium EDTA, natual flavor, vinamin E, beta carotene

Notes: Though it lists sugar as an ingredient, label says 0 sugars.

Braham & Murray Good Classic Mayonnaise
www.goodwebsite.us.com
Ingredients: water, cold pressed hemp seed oil (18%), rapeseed oil, sunflower oil, pasturised free range egg yolk (7%), white wine vinegar, sugar, prepared Dijon mustard (water, mustard seeds, distilled vinegar, salt), fruit fibre, salt, concentrated lemon juice, stabilizer, xanthan gum
Notes: GF, Vegetarian From UK.

Dickinson's Lemon Curd
www.dickinsonsfamily.com
Ingredients: sugar, water, eggs, butter (cream -from milk), salt, lemon juice concentrate, pectin, citric acid, natural flavor, sodium citrate, locust bean gum, yellow 5

Notes: 11g Sugar Other flavors available

Gourmet Temptations Mustard Blends Lemon Caper
www.gourmettemptations.com
Ingredients: Dijon mustard, distilled vinegar, water, mustard seed, white wine, sugar, spices, turmeric, capers, lemon puree (lemon juice concentrate, water, lemon pulp cells, lemon peel, lemon oil)

Notes: < 1g Sugar This makes an amazing salad dressing.

Jack Daniel's Old No. 7 Mustard
www.jackdanielsmustards.com
Ingredients: distilled vinegar, water, mustard seed, salt, spices, turmeric, natural flavors, old no. 7 whiskey

Notes: GF

Seggiano Raw Basil Pesto
www.seggiano.com
Ingredients: olive oil, cashew nuts, fresh Ligurian basil, sea salt, pine nuts

Notes: While this does have cashews, which can be problematic, it is the only pesto I have found without garlic.

Condiments - Continued

Westbrae Naturals Stoneground Mustard
www.westbrae.com
Ingredients: water, grain vinegar, organic mustard seeds, turmeric, salt, spices

Notes:

Westbrae Naturals Yellow Mustard
www.westbrae.com
Ingredients: water, grain vinegar, organic mustard seeds, turmeric, salt, spices

Notes:

Westbrae Naturals Dijon Mustard
www.westbrae.com
Ingredients: water, grain vinegar, organic mustard seeds, white wine vinegar, salt, spices

Notes:

Cookies/Bars

Remember, regardless of the ingredients, a cookie is still a cookie, which means sugar. If you should choose to indulge, be sure to keep the serving very small and infrequent. Also, as always, double-check the ingredients. We include this section to assist those who are searching for *any* possibilities for treats, not because they are a sure-thing for all FMer's.

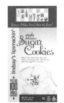

123 Gluten Free Lindsay's Lipsmacking Roll-out & Cut Sugar Cookies
www.123glutenfree.com

Ingredients: rice flour, sugar, tapioca flour, potato starch, natural flavoring, aluminum-free/corn-free baking powder (sodium acid pyrophosphate, baking soda, potato starch, monocalcium phosphate), salt

Notes: GF, WF, DF, CSF, PF, TNF, CF, EF, SF, Non-GMO, 8g Sugar

123 Gluten Free Sweet Goodness Pan Bars
www.123glutenfree.com

Ingredients: sugar, rice flour, tapioca flour, potato starch, baking soda, spices, aluminum-free/corn-free baking powder (sodium acid pyrophosphate, baking soda, potato starch, monocalcium phosphate), salt, xanthan gum

Notes: GF, WF, DF, CF, PF, TNF, CF, EF, SF, 14g Sugar Recipes on-line.

Alternative Baking Company Cinnamon Burst Cookie
www.alternativebaking.com

Ingredients: gluten-free flour (garbanzo bean flour, potato starch, tapioca flour, sorghum flour, fava bean flour), organic unrefined cane sugar, fruit juice and natural grain dextrins, palm oil, water, vanilla, natural tapioca & potato starches, natural spices, sea salt, aluminum-free baking powder, baking soda, sea salt, xanthan gum
Notes: GF, 19g Sugar Produced in a facility that also handles peanuts, tree nuts, and wheat.

Alternative Baking Company Lemon Dream Cookie
www.alternativebaking.com

Ingredients: gluten-free flour (garbanzo bean flour, potato starch, tapioca flour, sorghum flour, fava bean flour), organic unrefined cane sugar, fruit juice and natural grain dextrins, palm oil, water, natural tapioca & potato starches, vanilla, lemon extract, sea salt, aluminum-free baking powder, baking soda, sea salt, xanthan gum
Notes: GF, 19g Sugar Produced in a facility that also handles peanuts, tree nuts, and wheat.

Alternative Baking Company Pumpkin Delight Cookie
www.alternativebaking.com

Ingredients: gluten-free flour (garbanzo bean flour, potato starch, tapioca flour, sorghum flour, fava bean flour), organic unrefined cane sugar, pumpkin, fruit juice and natural grain dextrins, palm oil, water, natural tapioca & potato starches, vanilla, **natural spices**, sea salt, aluminum-free baking powder, baking soda, sea salt, xanthan gum
Notes: GF, 20g Sugar Produced in a facility that also handles peanuts, tree nuts, and wheat.

Amy's Shortbread Almond Cookie
www.amys.com

Ingredients: organic grade AA butter (organic cream, salt), almond flour, organic whole grain brown rice flour, organic evaporated cane juice, organic almonds, organic sorghum flour, organic almond extract

Notes: GF, SF, Kosher, 3g Sugar

Cookies/Bars - Continued

Andean Dream Quinoa Cookies Orange Essence
www.andeandream.com
Ingredients: organic royal quinoa flour, tapioca flour, non-hydrogenated palm fruit oil, raw sugar, sugar cane syrup, rice flour, organic quinoa pop grains, sodium bicarbonate (baking soda), natural orange extract (alcohol and corn free)
Notes: GF, CF, Vegan, 4g Sugar

Betsy's Best Bar None Cinnamon Cardamom
www.betsysbestbarnone.com
Ingredients: coconut nectar, pumpkin seed butter, almond butter, hemp, chia, quinoa, flax, coconut oil, cinnamon, sea salt, vanilla extract, cardamom

Notes: GF, SF, Vegan, Organic, Non-GMO, 8g Sugar

Deborah Kaye's Cookies - Oatmeal Walnut
www.deborahkayes.com
Ingredients: certified gluten free rolled oats, natural sucanuut, canola oil, natural walnuts, organic coconut, organic eggs, natural vanilla, sea salt, xanthan gum

Notes: GF, DF, CF, Non-GMO, 8g Sugar

Cherrybrook Kitchen Gluten Free Dreams Sugar Cookie Mix
www.cherrybrookkitchen.com
Ingredients: white rice flour, evaporated cane juice, potato starch, tapioca flour, non-alluminated baking powder, xanthan gum, sea salt

Notes: GF, DF, EF, TNF, PF, 7g Sugar

Liz Lovely Lemon-E Poppy Cookie
www.lizlovely.com
Ingredients: evaporated cane juice, white rice flour, water, potato starch, palm fruit oil, tapioca flour, lemon oil, poppy seeds vanilla extract, xanthan gum, sea salt, baking soda, sea salt, natural tocopherols (vitamin E)
Notes: WF, DF, EF, GF, Non-GMO, Vegan, 14g Sugar Free Shipping

Liz Lovely Snickerdoodle Cookie
www.lizlovely.com
Ingredients: rice flour, unrefined cane sugar, palm fruit oil, potato starch, Vermont well water, tapioca starch, cream of tartar, vanilla extract, baking soda, sea salt, xanthan gum, cinnamon

Notes: WF, DF, EF, GF, Non-GMO, Vegan, 13g Sugar Free Shipping

The No-Bake Cookie Company Almond Butter
www.thenobakecookieco.com
Ingredients: gluten free oats, sugar, non fat milk (vitamin A palmitate, Vitamin D3), natural almond butter, butter (pasteurized cream, salt), pure vanilla
Notes: GF, Sugars N/A Processed on shared equipment that processes peanuts

Cookies/Bars - Continued

Silly Yak Bakery Snickerdoodle Cookie

www.freshglutenfree.net

Ingredients: rice flower, potato starch, arrowroot starch, granulated sugar, butter, eggs, xanthan gum, cinnamon, cream of tartar, baking soda, salt

Notes: GF, 25g Sugar

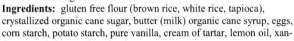

WOW Baking Company Lemonburst Cookie

www.wowbaking.com

Ingredients: gluten free flour (brown rice, white rice, tapioca), crystallized organic cane sugar, butter (milk) organic cane syrup, eggs, corn starch, potato starch, pure vanilla, cream of tartar, lemon oil, xanthan gum, baking soda, salt, cinnamon

Notes: WF, GF, 20g Sugar

Crackers

Blue Diamond Natural Almond Nut-Thins
www.bluediamond.com
Ingredients: rice flour, almonds, potato starch, salt, expeller pressed safflower oil, salt, natural almond flavor, natural butter flavor (contains milk)

Notes: GF, WF

Blue Diamond Natural Pecan Nut-Thins
www.bluediamond.com
Ingredients: rice flour, pecan meal, potato starch, salt, expeller pressed safflower oil, salt, natural pecan flavor, natural butter flavor (contains milk)

Notes: GF, WF

Edward & Sons Exotic Rice Toast
www.edwardandsons.org
Ingredients: red rice flour, natural tapioca starch, expeller-pressed palm oil, organic evaporated cane juice, flaxseed, salt, natural vitamin E oil (antioxidant -contains soy)

Notes: GF, WF, Vegan, < 1g Sugar

Glutino Gluten Free Crackers Multigrain
www.glutino.com
Ingredients: corn starch, white rice flour, organic palm oil, modified corn starch, dextrose, eggs, sunflower lecithin, buckwheat bran, salt, poppy seeds, guar gum, flax seeds, sodium bicarbonate, ammonium bicarbonate, rosemary extract
Notes: GF, 1g Sugar

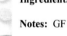
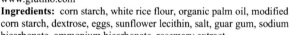

Glutino Gluten Free Crackers Original
www.glutino.com
Ingredients: corn starch, white rice flour, organic palm oil, modified corn starch, dextrose, eggs, sunflower lecithin, salt, guar gum, sodium bicarbonate, ammonium bicarbonate, rosemary extract

Notes: GF, 1g Sugar

Nabisco Gluten Free Rice Thins Original

www.snackworks.com
Ingredients: white rice flour, high oleic safflower oil, salt

Notes: GF

Creamers

Bailey's Coffee Creamer
www.baileyscreamers.com
Ingredients: water, sugar, cream, natural and artificial flavors, disodium phosphate, sodium caseinate, artificial color, salt, carageenan

Notes: GF, 5g Sugar

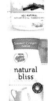

Coffee Mate Natural Bliss Creamer Cinnamon
www.naturalbliss.coffee-mate.com
Ingredients: nonfat milk, heavy cream, sugar, natural flavor

Notes: 5g Sugar Different flavors have different ingredients.

Coffee Mate Natural Bliss Creamer Sweet Cream
www.naturalbliss.coffee-mate.com
Ingredients: nonfat milk, heavy cream, sugar, natural flavor

Notes: 5g Sugar

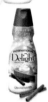

Coffee Mate Natural Bliss Creamer Vanilla
www.naturalbliss.coffee-mate.com
Ingredients: milk, cream, sugar, natural vanilla flavor

Notes: 5g Sugar

International Delight Creamer Pumpkin Pie Spice
www.internationaldelight.com
Ingredients: water, sugar, palm oil, contains 2% or less of each of the following: sodium caseinate (a milk derivative), dipotassium phosphate, natural and artificial flavors, mono and diglycerides, sodium stearcyl lactylate, polysorbate 60, carrageenan, salt
Notes: 6g Sugar Different flavors have different ingredients; some have corn syrup

Dressings

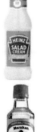

Heinz Salad Cream Original
www.heinz.com

Ingredients: spirit vinegar, canola oil, water, sugar, mustard, salt, egg yolks, modified corn starch, xantham gum, gar gum, colored with riboflavin

Notes: 3g Sugar

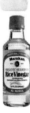

Marukan Organic Seasoned Rice Vinegar Dressing
www.marukan-usa.com

Ingredients: organic rice vinegar (water, organic rice), sugar (organic sugar), salt (sea salt)

Notes: GF, Non-GMO, 3g Sugar

Drinks

Glaceau Vitamin Water Zero
www.vitaminwater.com
Ingredients:

Notes: various flavors, check ingredients

Hansen's Natural Soda - Creamy Root Beer
www.hansens.com
Ingredients: pure triple filtered carbonated water, sugar, caramel color, natural spices of wintergreen, birch, anise, and sassafras, Tahitian vanilla extract, citric acid
,
Notes: 27g Sugar, several flavors available

Natural Brew - Root Beer
www.natural-brew.com
Ingredients: sparkling filtered water, sugar, natural flavors, bourbon vanilla extract, anise, licorice root, birch oil, wintergreen oil, caramel color, phosphoric acid

Notes: 41g Sugar, several flavors available

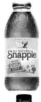

Sierra Mist
www.pepsicobeveragefacts.com
Ingredients: carbonated water, sugar, citric acid, natural flavor, potassium citrate

Notes: 25g Sugar

Snapple All Natural Lemon Tea
www.snapple.com
Ingredients: filtered water, sugar, citric acid, tea, natural flavors

Notes: 36g Sugar

Sobe GreenTea
www.sobe.com
Ingredients: filtered water, sugar, natural flavor, citric acid, ascorbic acid (vitamin C), gree tea extract, caramel color, reb A (purified stevia extract), guarana seed extract, panax ginseng root extract, rose hips extract
Notes: 21g Sugar in 8 ounces

Tazo
www.tazo.com
Ingredients: an infusion of (water, green tea, lemongrass, spearmint, lemon verbena, natural flavor), cane sugar, citric acid

Notes: 18g Sugar

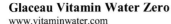

Flours & Meals

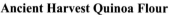

123 Gluten Free Olivia's Outstanding Multi-Purpose Flour Mix
www.123glutenfree.com
Ingredients: rice flour, potato starch, tapioca starch, xanthan gum, niacin (vitamin B3), reduced iron, thiamin mononitrate (vitamin B2), folic acid (vitamin B9)

Ancient Harvest Quinoa Flour
www.quinoa.net
Ingredients: quinoa

Notes: GF, WF, Non-GMO, 1g Sugar

Arrowhead Mills Buckwheat Flour
www.arrowheadmills.com
Ingredients: organic buckwheat flour

Notes: GF, WF, DF, Vegetarian, < 1g Sugar

Arrowhead Mills Millet Flour
www.arrowheadmills.com
Ingredients: organic wholegrain millet flour

Notes: GF, WF, DF, Vegetarian

Arrowhead Mills White Rice Flour
www.arrowheadmills.com
Ingredients: organic white rice flour

Notes: GF, WF, DF, Vegetarian

Arrowhead Mills Flax Seed Meal
www.arrowheadmills.com
Ingredients: organic flax seed

Notes:

Arrowhead Mills Organic Oat Flour
www.arrowheadmills.com
Ingredients: certified organic whole grain oat flour

Notes: WF, DF, Vegetarian

Flours & Meals - Continued

Arrowhead Mills White Rice Flour
www.arrowheadmills.com
Ingredients: organic white rice flour

Notes: WF, DF, Vegetarian

Bob's Red Mill Almond Meal
www.bobsredmill.com
Ingredients: blanched almonds

Notes: GF, 1g Sugar Manufactured in a facility that also uses soy, wheat.

Bob's Red Mill Amaranth Flour
www.bobsredmill.com
Ingredients: whole grain amaranth

Notes: GF, Manufactured in a facility that also uses soy, wheat.

Bob's Red Mill Buckwheat Flour
www.bobsredmill.com
Ingredients: whole grain organic buckwheat

Notes: GF Manufactured in a facility that also uses soy, wheat.

Bob's Red Mill Flax Seed Meal
www.bobsredmill.com
Ingredients: whole ground flaxseed

Notes: GF Manufactured in a facility that also uses soy, wheat.

Bob's Red Mill Potato Flour
www.bobsredmill.com
Ingredients: potato

Notes: GF Manufactured in a facility that also uses soy, wheat.

Bob's Red Mill Hazelnut Flour
www.bobsredmill.com
Ingredients: hazelnuts

Notes: GF, 1g Sugar Manufactured in a facility that also uses nuts and soy.

Flours & Meals - Continued

Bob's Red Mill Gluten Free Oat Flour
www.bobsredmill.com
Ingredients: gluten free whole grain oats

Notes: GF, WF, DF

Bob's Red Mill Quinoa Flour
www.bobsredmill.com
Ingredients: organic whole grain quinoa

Notes: GF

Bob's Red Mill Sweet White Rice Flour
www.bobsredmill.com
Ingredients: sweet white rice

Notes: GF, 1g Sugar

Bob's Red Mill Tapioca Flour
www.bobsredmill.com
Ingredients: tapioca

Notes: GF, Good substitute for corn starch

Bob's Red Mill Teff Flour
www.bobsredmill.com
Ingredients: whole grain teff

Notes: GF, Ancient North African cereal grass.

Bob's Red Mill White Rice Flour
www.bobsredmill.com
Ingredients: white rice

Notes: GF

Dawd & Roger California Almond Flour
www.dawdandrodgers.com
Ingredients: 100% ground almonds

Notes: GF, WF, 3g Sugar

Flours & Meals - Continued

Dawd & Rodger Chia Omega Flour
www.dawdandrodgers.com
Ingredients: chai grain, rose tapioca flour, millet flour, chestnut flour, xanthan gum

Notes: GF, Sugar grams unavailable

Dawd & Rodger Chestnut Flour
www.dawdandrodgers.com
Ingredients: 100% ground chestnut

Notes: GF, WF, 3g Sugar

Grains - Listed By Grain

Bob's Red Mill Buckwheat Groats

www.bobsredmill.com
Ingredients: organic buckwheat groats

Notes: GF, 1g Sugar Manufactured in a facility that also uses soy, wheat.

Eden Organic Buckwheat

www.edenfoods.com
Ingredients: organic hulled buckwheat

Notes: GF, WF, Non-GMO

Bob's Red Mill Flaxseed

www.bobsredmill.com
Ingredients: whole brown flaxseeds

Notes:

Bob's Red Mill Golden Flaxseed

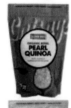

www.bobsredmill.com.com
Ingredients: golden flaxseed

Notes:

Alter Eco Organic Royal Pearl Quinoa

www.alterecofoods.com
Ingredients: 100% organic royal white quinoa

Notes: GF, Non-GMO, Vegan

Alter Eco Royal Rainbow Quinoa

www.alterecofoodscom
Ingredients: 100% organic royal white quinoa, 100% organic royal red quinoa, 100% organic royal black quinoa,

Notes: GF, Non-GMO, Vegan

Alter Eco Royal RedQuinoa

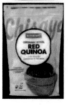

www.alterecofoodscom
Ingredients: 100% organic royal red quinoa

Notes: GF, Non-GMO, Vegan

Grains - Continued

Ancient Harvest Organic Inca Red Quinoa
www.quinoa.net
Ingredients: organic red quinoa

Notes: GF, 3.2g Sugar

Ancient Harvest Organic Inca Traditional Quinoa
www.quinoa.net
Ingredients: organic quinoa

Notes: GF, 1g Sugar

Eden Organic Quinoa
www.edenfoods.com
Ingredients: organic quinoa

Notes: GF, WF, Non-GMO, 1g Sugar

Eden Organic Quinoa
www.edenfoods.com
Ingredients: organic red quinoa

Notes: GF, WF, Non-GMO

Tru Roots Whole Grain Quinoa
www.truroots.com
Ingredients: organic quinoa

Notes: GF, 4g Sugar

Tru Roots Sprouted Quinoa
www.truroots.com
Ingredients: organic quinoa

Notes: GF, 4g Sugar

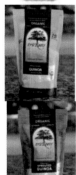

Woodstock Farms Organic White Quinoa

Ingredients: organic white quinoa

Notes: Non-GMO, 1g Sugar

Grains - Continued

Alter Eco Organic Hom Mali Jasmine Rice

www.alterecofoods.com
Ingredients: organic hom mali jasmine rice

Notes: GF, Non-GMO

La Preferida Organic Long Grain White Rice

www.lapreferida.com
Ingredients: organicily grown US long grain white rice

Notes: GF

Lotus Organic Jade Pearl Rice

www.lotusfoods.com
Ingredients: organic rice, wildcrafted bamboo extract

Notes: Non-GMO, FT, Kosher

Lotus Organic Mekong Flower Rice

www.lotusfoods.com
Ingredients: **100%** organic white rice

Notes: Non-GMO, FT, Kosher

Lundberg California Sushi Rice

www.lundberg.com
Ingredients: organic California sushi rice

Notes: GF, Kosher, Non-GMO, Vegan

Lundberg California White Jasmine Rice

www.lundberg.com
Ingredients: organic white California jasmine rice

Notes: GF, Kosher, Non-GMO, Vegan

Lundberg Long Grain Organic White Rice

www.lundberg.com
Ingredients: organic white long grain rice

Notes: GF, Kosher, Non-GMO, Vegan

Grains - Continued

Shirakiku Calrose Rice

Ingredients: medium grain Japanese-style rice

Notes:

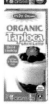

Let's Do...Organic Tapioca Pearls
www.edwardandsons.com
Ingredients: organic tapioca

Notes: GF

Let's Do...Organic Tapioca Granules
www.edwardandsons.com
Ingredients: organic tapioca, citric acid

Notes: GF

Ice Cream/Frozen Yogurt/Gelato

Obviously, ice cream will have sugar, but as with other treat items listed, this is for informational purposes. Only you know your tolerance level for sugars. Our hope is to give options.

Alden's Organic Ice Cream (Blackberry, Strawberry, Vanilla Bean, Butter Brittle)
www.aldensicecream.com
Ingredients: organic milk, organic cream, organic cane sugar, organic tapioca syrup, organic vanilla extract, milk mineral (calcium), organic tapioca starch, non-GMP soy lecithin, guar gum, locust bean gum, xanthan gum, natural flavor, annatto extract (color)
Notes: Organic, Non-GMO, Kosher, 14g Sugar (vanilla)

Ben & Jerry's Vanilla Ice Cream
www.benjerry.com
Ingredients: cream, skim milk, liquid sugar (sugar, water), water, egg yolks, fair trade certified ™ vanilla extract, sugar, guar gum, carrageenan
Notes: 20g Sugar

Breyers Vanilla Ice Cream
www.breyers.com
Ingredients: milk, cream, sugar, tara gum, natural flavor

Notes: 14g Sugar

Cefiore Non-Fat Frozen Yogurt - Original Tart
www.cefiore.com
Ingredients: water, skim milk, sucrose, maltodextrin (soluble dietary fiber), whey, egg yokes, citric acid, natural flavor, stabilizer (locust bean gum), guar gum, carrageenun, yogurt culture, natural lemon juice powder

Cefiore Non-Fat Frozen Yogurt - Strawberry
www.cefiore.com
Ingredients: water, sucrose, strawberries, skim milk, strawberry puree, maltodextrin (soluble dietary fiber), whey, egg yokes, citric acid, stabilizer (locust bean gum, guar gum), carrageenun, yogurt culture, natural lemon juice powder
Notes: Sugar Grams Unavailable

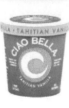

Ciao Bella Tahitian Vanilla Gelato
www.ciaobellagelato.com
Ingredients: milk, cream, organic evaporated cane juice, non-fat dry milk, tapioca syrup, vanilla extract, gar gum, locust bean gum, carageenan, vanilla bean specks

Notes: 18g Sugar

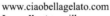

Ice Cream/Frozen Yogurt/Gelato-Cont.

Ciao Bella Matcha Green Tea Gelato
www.ciaobellagelato.com
Ingredients: cream, skim milk, liquid sugar (sugar, water), water, egg yolks, fair milk, cream, organic evaporated cane juice, non-fat dry milk, tapioca syrup, green tea, gar gum, locust bean gum, carageenan

Notes: 17.5g Sugar

Ciao Bella Triple Espresso Gelato
www.ciaobellagelato.com
Ingredients: milk, cream, organic evaporated cane juice, non-fat dry milk, tapioca syrup, espresso concentrate, coffee concentrate, Napoli coffee, gar gum, locust bean gum, carageenan

Notes: 16g Sugar

Double Rainbow French Vanilla
www.doublerainbow.com
Ingredients: cream, milk, cane sugar, egg yolks, natural vanilla flavor, carob bean gum, guar gum

Notes: 22g Sugar

Goldbaum's Cones
www.goldbaums.com
Ingredients: potato starch, sugar, tapioca starch, palm oil(GMO free), dietary fibers, emulsifier (lecithin), cocoa powder, salt, stabilizer (xanthan gum), baking soda, natural vanilla
Notes: GF, Kosher, GMO-free, Vegan
This is as close as we have found for ice cream cones.

Graeter's Vanilla Ice Cream
www.graeters.com
Ingredients: organic milk, organic cream, organic cane sugar, organic tapioca syrup, organic vanilla cream, milk, cane sugar, corn sugar, eggs, vanilla bean, vanilla extract, guar gum, locust bean gum

Notes: 24g Sugar

Haagen-Dazs Vanilla Bean Ice Cream (Vanilla)
www.haagendazs.com
Ingredients: cream, skim milk, sugar, egg yolks, ground vanilla beans, vanilla extract

Notes: 17g Sugar

Julie's Organic Ice Cream Blackberry
www.juliesorganic.com
Ingredients: fresh organic cream, organic skim milk, organic evaporated cane juice, organic egg yolks, organic vanilla extract, carob bean gum, guar gum, blackberry

Notes: 21g Sugar

Ice Cream/Frozen Yogurt/Gelato-Cont.

Julie's Organic Ice Cream Caramel
www.juliesorganic.com
Ingredients: fresh organic cream, organic skim milk, organic evaporated cane juice, organic egg yolks, organic vanilla extract, carob bean gum, guar gum, caramel

Notes: 22g Sugar

Julie's Organic Ice Cream Vanilla
www.juliesorganic.com
Ingredients: fresh organic cream, organic skim milk, organic evaporated cane juice, organic egg yolks, organic vanilla extract, carob bean gum, guar gum

Notes: 18g Sugar

Julie's Organic Gluten Free Lemon Yogurt Sandwich Cookies
www.juliesorganic.com
Ingredients: Yogurt-org cultured skim milk, org cane sugar, org tapioca syrup, org cream, fructan (naturaflora soluble fiber), org lemon juice concentrate, org tapioca starch, citric acid, natural flavor, org guar gum, org locust bean gum, org turmeric (for color), contains live active yogurt and probiotic cultures **Gluten Free Vanilla Cookie-**org rice flour, org cane sugar, org corn starch, org butter, org potato starch, org eggs, org vanilla baking soda, salt, 21g Sugar

La Loos Goats Milk Cappracino Ice Cream
www.laloos.com
Ingredients: goat milk, sugar, Italian espresso roast coffee bean, pure vanilla, egg yolks, locust bean gum, guar gum, carrageenan

Notes: 14g sugar

La Loos Goats Milk Ice Cream Vanilla Snowflake
www.laloos.com
Ingredients: goat milk, sugar, egg yolks, pure vanilla, locust bean gum, guar gum, carrageenan

Notes: 14g sugar

Stonyfield Cream Caramel Lowfat Frozen Yogurt
www.www.stonyfield.com
Ingredients: cultured pasteurized organic non-fat milk, naturally milled organic sugar, organic rice syrup, organic whey protein concentrate, organic vanilla flavor, organic carob bean gum, organic guar gum, organic vanilla bean specks
Notes: 25g Sugar

Stonyfield Gotta Have Vanilla Frozen Yogurt
www.stonyfield.com
Ingredients: cultured pasteurized organic non-fat milk, naturally milled organic sugar, organic rice syrup, organic whey protein concentrate, organic vanilla flavor, organic carob bean gum, organic guar gum, organic vanilla bean specks
Notes: 19g Sugar

Ice Cream/Frozen Yogurt/Gelato-Cont.

Straus Family Creamery Organic Raspberry
www.strausfamilycreamery.com
Ingredients: pasteurized organic cream and organic nonfat milk, organic sugar, organic raspberry puree, organic egg yolk, organic vanilla, extract
Notes: GF, Non-GMO, Kosher, 19g Sugar Their other flavors have dark brown sugar.

Three Twins Organic Ice Cream Dad's Cardamom
www.threetwinsicecream.com
Ingredients: organic milk, organic cream, organic evaporated cane juice, organic egg yolks, organic nonfat milk, organic vanilla extract, organic cardamom
Notes: 17g Sugar

Three Twins Organic Ice Cream Fair Trade Vanilla Bean Speck
www.threetwinsicecream.com
Ingredients: organic milk, organic cream, organic fair trade evaporated cane juice, organic egg yolks, organic nonfat milk, organic fair trade vanilla beans
Notes: FT, 15g Sugar

Three Twins Organic Ice Cream Madagascar Vanilla
www.threetwinsicecream.com
Ingredients: organic milk, organic cream, organic evaporated cane juice, organic egg yolks, organic nonfat milk, organic vanilla extract

Notes: 15g Sugar

Three Twins Organic Ice Cream Sea Salted Caramel
www.threetwinsicecream.com
Ingredients: organic milk, organic cream, organic evaporated cane juice, caramel (organic sugar, organic cream, organic non fat milk, organic tapioca syrup, organic caramelized sugar, sea salt), organic egg yolks, organic nonfat milk, organic vanilla extract,
Notes: 17g Sugar

Jams/Jellies

Note: Made from fruit juice / pieces, usually with sugar, so these should be limited to extremely small amounts. Also, look for locally available low/no sugar jars.

Crofter's Premium Spread Strawberry Organic
www.croftersorganic.com
Ingredients: organic strawberries, organic cane sugar, natural apple pectin, ascorbic acid (vitamin C), citric acid

Notes: WF, GF, Non-GMO, 8g Sugar

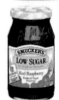

Smucker's Low Sugar Red Raspberry Preserves
www.smuckers.com
Ingredients: red raspberries, sugar, water, fruit pectin, citric acid, locust bean gum, potassium, sorbate added as a preservative, calcium chloride

Notes: 5g Sugar

Smucker's Low Sugar Strawberry Preserves
www.smuckers.com
Ingredients: strawberries, sugar, water, fruit pectin, citric acid, locust bean gum, potassium sorbate added as a preservative, calcium chloride, red 40

Notes: 5g Sugar

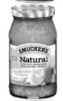

Smucker's Natural Orange Marmalade
www.smuckers.com
Ingredients: sugar, orange juice, orange peel, water, fruit pectin, citric acid

Notes: 10g Sugar

Smucker's Natural Red Raspberry Fruit Spread
www.smuckers.com
Ingredients: red raspberries, sugar, fruit pectin, citric acid

Notes: 10g Sugar

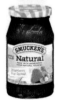

Smucker's Natural Strawberry Fruit Spread
www.smuckers.com
Ingredients: strawberries, sugar, fruit pectin, citric acid

Notes: 10g Sugar

Meats

Boar's Head All Natural Uncured Ham
www.boarshead.com
Ingredients:

Notes: GF, DF, 1g Sugar

Hormel Natural Choice Cooked Deli Ham
www.hormel.com
Ingredients: ham, water, salt, turbinado sugar, natural flavoring, lactic acid starter culture (not from milk)

Notes: GF, 1g sugar

Hormel Natural Choice Deli Roast Beef
www.hormel.com
Ingredients: beef, water, salt, turbinado sugar, baking soda

Notes: GF

Hormel Natural Choice Original Uncured Bacon
www.hormel.com
Ingredients: pork, water, salt, turbinado sugar, seasoning (cultured celery juice powder, sea salt)

Notes:

Hormel Natural Choice Oven Roasted Turkey
www.hormel.com
Ingredients: turkey breast meat, water, salt, potato starch, turbinado sugar, rice starch, carrageenan (from seaweed), baking soda, celery juice powder, lactic acid starter culture (not from milk).

Notes: GF, 1g Sugar

Hormel Natural Choice Rotisserie Style Deli Chicken Brest
www.hormel.com
Ingredients: chicken breast meat, water, salt, turbinado sugar, carrageenan, natural cure (celery powder, sea salt, lactic acid starter culture), baking soda (sodium bicarbonate)
Notes: GF

Hormel Natural Choice Smoked Deli Ham
www.hormel.com
Ingredients: ham, water, salt, turbinado sugar, natural flavoring, lactic acid starter culture (not from milk)

Notes: GF, 3g Sugar

Meats - Continued

Oberto All Natural Bacon Jerky
www.oberto.com
Ingredients: bacon, water, sea salt, sugar, natural flavoring

Notes: GF, 1g Sugar

Shelton's Uncured Chicken Franks
www.sheltons.com
Ingredients: chicken meat, water, sea salt, spices, potato starch

Notes:

Shelton's Uncured Turkey Franks
www.sheltons.com
Ingredients: turkey meat, water, sea salt, spices, potato starch

Notes: Also available in a smoked version.

Stryker Farm Uncured Pork Hot Dog
www.strykerfarm.com
Ingredients: pork, water, sea salt, maple syrup, spices

Notes:

Medications

While some of these may contain sorbitol, I have had no problem taking them and many report using them.

Advil Liqui-Gels
www.advil.com
Inactive Ingredients: coconut oil, FD&C green no. 3, gelatin, lecithin, light mineral oil, pharmaceutical ink, polyethylene glycol, potassium hydroxide, purified water, sorbitan, sorbitol
Notes: While this contains sorbitol, I can tolerate it if I do not take more than one dose.

Benadryl Allergy Liqui Gels
www.benadryl.com
Ingredients: dephenhydramine, gelatin, glycerin, polyethylene glycol, purified water , sorbitol

Notes:

MiraLax
www.miralax.com
Ingredients: polyethylene glycol

Notes: GF Be sure it is completely dissolved before drinking!

Ricola Original Natural Herb Cough Drops
www.ricola.com
Ingredients: menthol, color (caramel), extract of Ricola's herb mixture (elder, horehound, hyssop, lemon balm, linden flowers, mallow, peppermint, sage, thyme, wild thyme), peppermint oil, starch syrup, sugar

Notes: 3.2g Sugar

Milk

Obviously, unless you are lactose intolerant or vegan, you have plenty of cow and goat milk options. However, if one of these are a concern, or if you simply wish to expand your selection a bit, this category will offer some available options.

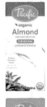

Pacific Organic Unsweetened Almond Original
www.pacificfoods.com
Ingredients: organic almond base (filtered water, organic almonds), organic rice starch, sea salt, organic vanilla, natural flavor, carrageenan, riboflavin (B2), vitamin A palmitate, vitamin D2,

Notes: GF, WF, SF, DF, YF, Kosher, Vegan, Non-GMO

Pacific Organic Oat Original
www.pacificfoods.com
Ingredients: filtered water, organic oats, organic oat bran, tricalcium phosphate, sea salt, gellan gum, riboflavin (B2), vitamin A palmitate, vitamin D2
Notes: WF, DF, SF, YF, Kosher, Vegan, Non-GMO, 19g Sugar

Pacific Organic Oat Vanilla
www.pacificfoods.com
Ingredients: filtered water, organic oats, organic oat bran, tricalcium phosphate, natural vanilla flavor with other natural flavors, sea salt, gellan gum, riboflavin (B2), vitamin A palmitate, vitamin D2

Notes: WF, DF, SF, YF, Kosher, Vegan, Non-GMO, 20g Sugar

Silk Almondmilk Original
www.silk.com
Ingredients: almond milk (filtered water, almonds), cane sugar, sea salt, locust bean gum, sunflower lecithin, gellan gum

Notes: GF, DF, SF, EF, CSF, Non-GMO, 7g Sugar

Silk Almondmilk Vanilla
www.silk.com
Ingredients: almond milk (filtered water, almonds), cane sugar, sea salt, natural flavor, locust bean gum, sunflower lecithin, gellan gum

Notes: GF, DF, SF, EF, CSF, Non-GMO, 16g Sugar

Silk Almondmilk Unsweetened Vanilla
www.silk.com
Ingredients: almond milk (filtered water, almonds), sea salt, natural flavor, locust bean gum, sunflower lecithin, gellan gum

Notes: GF, DF, SF, EF, CSF, Non-GMO

Milk - Continued

Silk Almondmilk Light Vanilla
www.silk.com
Ingredients: almond milk (filtered water, almonds), cane sugar, sea salt, locust bean gum, natural flavor, sunflower lecithin, gellan gum

Notes: GF, DF, SF, EF, CSF, Non-GMO, 11g Sugar

Sunflower Dream Sunflower Drink Unsweetened
www.tastethedream.com
Ingredients: sunflower base (flitered water, sunflower kernels, sunflower lecithin, citric acid), tricalcium phosphate, tapioca starch, sea salt, xanthan gum, natural flavors, guar gum, carrageenan, vitamin E (D-alpha tocopheryl acetate), vitamin A palmitate, folic acid, vitamin D2
Notes: GF, DF, Kosher, Vegan, Non-GMO

Miscellaneous

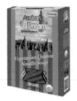

Andean Dream Vegetarian Quinoa Noodle Soup
www.andeandream.com
Ingredients: organic pre-cooked white quinoa, organic quinoa-rice noodles (some with organic natural colors from spinach, beet root, and turmeric), also contains organic precooked red quinoa

Notes: GF, CF, Vegan, < 1g Sugar

Asafetida
Ingredients: varies by brand, some are cut with wheat, be sure to read ingredients

Brand not Available

Notes: Also known as Hing. Has an onion and garlic flavor when cooked in dishes. Don't try it straight/dry, it tastes awful and leaves a horrid lingering aftertaste. *Warning...unsafe for use in pregnancy or breast feeding, associated with miscarriage or bleeding disorders in infants. Check drug interactions.*

dōTerra Peppermint Beadlets
www.doterra.com
Ingredients: peppermint essential oil, fatty acid of coconut, gelatin

Notes:

Goldbaum's Crispy 'N Crunchy Gluten-Free Chow Mein Noodles
www.goldbaums.com
Ingredients: palm kernel, vegetable oil, tapioca starch, potato starch, pasteurized egg white, salt, spices (sweet pepper)

Notes:

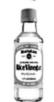

Marukan Organic Rice Vinegar
www.marukan-usa.com
Ingredients: rice vinegar (water, rice)

Notes: Non-GMO

Nestle Premier White Morsels
www.verybestbaking.com
Ingredients: sugar, fractionated palm kernel oil, skim milk, whey, milkfat, hydrogenated palm oil, soy lecithin - an emulsifier, natural and artificial flavors

Notes: 7g Sugar

Nut Butters

Adams 100% Natural Peanut Butter
www.adamspeanutbutter.com
Ingredients: **peanuts,** contains 1% or less of salt

Notes: 1g Sugar
Also available in organic

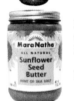

Artisana 100% Organic Raw Almond Butter
www.artisana.com
Ingredients: 100% organic raw almonds

Notes: Vegan, Kosher, 1g Sugar Made in a facility that processes tree nuts, but does not process any peanuts, dairy, gluten, or soy.

MaraNatha Sunflower Seed Butter
www.sunbutter.com
Ingredients: roasted sunflower kernel seeds, sea salt

Notes:

Nuttzo 7 Nut and Seed Butter
www.gonutzo.com
Ingredients: organic peanuts, organic cashews, organic almonds, organic flax sees, organic Brazilian nuts, organic hazelnuts, organic sunflower seeds, sea salt
Notes: 1g Sugar Jars are PET BFP-Free plastic.

Nuttzo 7 Nut and Seed Butter - Peanut Free
www.gonutzo.com
Ingredients: organic cashews, organic almonds, organic Brazil nuts, organic flax seeds, organic hazelnuts, organic chia seeds, organic pumpkin seeds, sea salt

Notes: PF, 1g Sugar Jars are PET BFP-Free plastic.

Skippy Natural Peanut Butter
www.peanutbutter.com
Ingredients: roasted peanuts, sugar, palm oil, salt

Notes: 3g Sugar No preservatives, artificial flavors, or colors.
Why buy peanut butter with oil and sugar added?

Sunbutter Creamy
www.sunbutter.com
Ingredients: sunflower seed**,** sugar, mono-diglycerides to prevent separation, salt, natural mixed tocopherols to preserve freshness

Notes: PF, TNF, GF, 3g Sugar

Nut Butters - continued

Sunbutter Natural
www.sunbutter.com
Ingredients: sunflower seed, flaxseed, evaporated cane syrup, salt, natural mixed tocopherols to preserve freshness

Notes: PF, TNF, GF, 3g Sugar

Sunbutter Organic

www.sunbutter.com
Ingredients: organic sunflower seed

Notes: PF, TNF, GF, 1g Sugar

Trader Joe's Almond Butter
www.traderjoes.com
Ingredients: dry roasted almonds

Notes: MSGF, Non-GMO, 2g Sugar Made on equipment shared with peanuts, tree nuts and soy.

Woodstock Farms Raw Almond Butter
www.woodstock-foods.com
Ingredients: raw unblanced almonds

Notes: Non-GMO, Vegan, 2g Sugar May contain trace amounts of peanuts, tree nuts, and seeds.

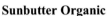

Pancake Mix

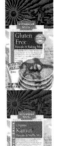

Arrowhead Mills Gluten Free Pancake and Baking Mix

www.arrowheadmills.com

Ingredients: organic white rice flour, organic potato starch, tapioca starch, baking powder (monocalcium phosphate, sodium bicarbonate, corn starch), organic whole grain yellow corn flour, natural flavor, sea salt, organic cinnamon

Notes: GF, WF, 1g Sugar

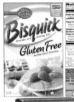

Arrowhead Mills Kamut Pancake and Waffle Mix

www.arrowheadmills.com

Ingredients: organic whole grain kamut flour, organic whole grain oat flour, organic soymilk powder, paking powder (monocalcium phosphate, sodium bicarbonate, corn starch), sea salt

Notes: GF

Bisquick Gluten Free Pancake and Baking Mix

www.bettycrocker.com

Ingredients: rice flour, sugar, levening (baking soda, sodium aluminum phospahate)

Notes: GF, WF, 3g Sugar

Cherrybrook Kitchen Gluten Free Dreams Pancake and Waffle Mix

www.cherrybrookkitchen.com

Ingredients: white rice flour, evaporated cane juice, potato starch, non-alluminated baking powder, tapioca starch, all natural vanilla flavor, sea salt, xanthan gum

Notes: GF, WF, PF, DF, TNF, EF, Vegan, 4g Sugar

White Pine Products Buckwheat Pancakes

www.whitepine.us.com

Ingredients: organic certified gluten-free buckwheat flour, organic evaporated cane juice, aluminum free non-GMO baking powder, kosher salt

Notes: GF, Non-GMO, Sugar grams unavailable

Pasta

A Taste of Thai Rice Noodles
www.atasteofthai.com
Ingredients: rice flour, water

Notes: GF, MSGF

Ancient Harvest Quinoa Pasta
www.quinoa.net
Ingredients: organic quinoa flour, organic corn flour

Notes: GF, Non-GMO, contains corn

Andean Dream Organic Pasta
www.andeandream.com
Ingredients: organic rice flour, organic quinoa flour

Notes: GF, CF, Kosher, 3g Sugar

Annie Chun's Maifun Rice Noodles
www.anniechun.com
Ingredients: rice flour, water

Notes: GF, WF

Annie Chun's Pad Thai Rice Noodles
www.anniechun.com
Ingredients: rice flour, water

Notes: GF, WF

DeBoles Gluten Free Rice Spaghetti Style Pasta
www.deboles.com
Ingredients: rice flour, rice bran extract

Notes: GF, WF

KaMe All Natural Rice Sticks - Vermicelli
www.kame.com
Ingredients: rice, water

Notes:

Pasta - Continued

King Soba Organic 100% Buckwheat Gluten-Free Noodles

www.kingsoba.com

Ingredients: organic buckwheat flour, water

Notes: GF, WF, 1g Sugar

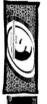

King Soba Organic Sweet Potato & Buckwheat Gluten-Free Noodles

www.kingsoba.com

Ingredients: organic buckwheat flour, organic sweet potato (5%), water

Notes: GF, WF, < 1g Sugar

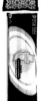

King Soba Organic Thai Rice Gluten-Free Noodles

www.kingsoba.com

Ingredients: organic thai rice flour, water

Notes: GF, WF, Non-GMO, Vegan, < 1g Sugar

Pasta Loioco (fusilli, macaroni, penne rigate, rigatoni, long pasta, spaghetti, fettuccini)

www.pastaglutenfree.net

Ingredients: rice flour, potato flour, xanthan gum, eggs, water, salt

Notes: GF, WF

Rustichella d'Abruzzo Organic Rice Penne Rigate

Ingredients: organic rice flour, water

Notes: GF, 1g Sugar

Sun Luck Maifun Rice Sticks (Phad Thai Rice Sticks)

Ingredients: rice flour, corn starch, water

Notes:

Thai Kitchen Stir-Fry Rice Noodles

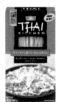

www.thaikitchen.com

Ingredients: rice flour, water

Notes:

Pasta Meals

Ancient Harvest Organic Mac & Cheese

www.ancientharvestquinoa.com

Ingredients: gluten-free pasta (corn flour, quinoa flour), cheese sauce mix (whey, maltodextrin [from corn], cheddar cheese [pasteurized milk, cheese cultures, salt, enzymes], corn startch, salt, natural flavors[from milk], sodium phosphate, annatto extract [color])

Notes: GF, Non-GMO, 4g Sugar

Annie's Rice Pasta & Cheddar Macaroni & Cheese

www.annies.com

Ingredients: rice pasta (rice flour), cheddar cheese (cultured pasteurized milk, salt, non-animal enzymes), whey, buttermilk, salt, cream, natural flavor, natural sodium phosphate, annatto extract for natural color,

Notes: GF, Non-GMO, 4g Sugar

Annie's Rice Shells and Creamy White Cheddar

www.annies.com

Ingredients: rice pasta shells (rice flour), cheddar cheese (cultured pasteurized milk, salt, non-animal enzymes), whey butter, nonfat milk, salt, sodium phosphate

Notes: GF, Non-GMO, 4g Sugar

Pasta Loioco Cheese Manicotti

www.pastaglutenfree.net

Ingredients: ricotta cheese, mozzarella cheese, parmesan cheese, rice flour, potato flour, tapioca starch, powder milk, xanthan gum, eggs, water, salt

Notes: GF

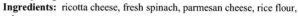

Pasta Loioco Gnocchi w/Spinach and Ricotta Cheese

www.pastaglutenfree.net

Ingredients: ricotta cheese, fresh spinach, parmesan cheese, rice flour, salt, pepper

Notes: GF, 1g Sugar

Potatoes

Bob's Red Mill Creamy Potato Flakes

www.bobsredmill.com

Ingredients: dehydrated potatoes

Notes:

Kroger Country Style Hash Browns

Ingredients: potatoes, dextrose, disodium dihydrogen pyrophosphate (to preserve color)

,
Notes:

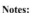

Ore Ida Simply Olive Oil and Sea Salt Country Style French Fries

www.oreida.com

Ingredients: potatoes, vegetable oil (olive oil, canola, sunflower, and/or cottonseed oils), sea salt, dextrose, citric acid (to promote color retention)

Notes:

Ore Ida Simply Olive Oil and Sea Salt Homestyle Wedges

www.oreida.com

Ingredients: potatoes, vegetable oil (olive oil, canola, sunflower, and/or cottonseed oils), sea salt, dextrose, citric acid (to promote color retention)

Notes:

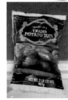

Trader Joe's Potato Tots

www.traderjoes.com

Ingredients: potatoes, vegetable oil (soybean/canola), salt, dextrose, citric acid to maintain color

,
Notes: MSGF, Non-GMO

Powders

Dr. Bernd Friedlander Protein Hydrate Collagen Peptide
www.zebraorganics.com
Ingredients:
,
Notes:

Garden of Life Raw Protein Powder
www.gardenoflife.com
Ingredients: Organic raw sprout blend: sprouted brown rice protein, amaranth sprout, quinoa sprout, millet sprout, buckwheat sprout, garbanzo bean sprout, lentil sprout, adzuki bean sprout, flax seed sprout, pumpkin seed sprout, chia seed sprout, sesame seed sprout **Other** **Ingredients:** raw natural vanilla flavor, organic stevia (leaf), brewers yeast, lactobacillus bulgaricus, natto (contains fermented soy

Notes: GF, DF, SF, Vegan, Non-GMO Some FMer's report this as okay, I have not tried it.

Nutiva Hemp Protein
www.storenutiva.com
Ingredients: organic hemp protein
,
Notes: DF, Non-GMO, 1g Sugar
Go to their Facebook page and like them, you can receive a single-use $10 coupon.

Snacks

Alive & Radiant Foods Kale Krunch OrganicPerfectly Plain
www.blessingaliveandradiantfoods.com
Ingredients: organic kale, organic pumpkin seeds,k organic lemon juice, organic chia seeds, organic extra virgin olive oil, Himalayan crystal salt
Notes:

Brothers-All-Natural Strawberry and Banana Crisps
www.brothersallnatural.com
Ingredients: 100% freeze-dried strawberries and bananas

Notes: GF, SF, DF, PF, TNF, Non GMO, Vegan, Kosher, 6g Sugar

Earth's Best Organic Banana Blueberry
www.earthsbest.com
Ingredients: organic bananas, organic blueberry puree, citric acid, vitamin A palmitate, mixed tocopherols (vitamin E), zinc sulfate, ascorbic acid
Notes: Kosher, 18g Sugar
While this is technically baby food, it makes a great, handy snack.

Earth's Best Organic Fruit Yogurt Smoothie
www.earthsbest.com
Ingredients: organic bananas, organic strawberries, organic yogurt (organic cultured pasteurized milk), water, calcium citrate malate, ascorbic acid (vitamin C), citric acid, vitamin D

Notes: Kosher, 15g Sugar

Go Raw Simple Granola
www.goraw.com
Ingredients: organic buckwheat groats, sprouted organic flax seed
,
Notes: GF, WF, TNF, 1g Sugar Maker suggests adding your own choice of nuts, fruits, etc. to this product.

Happy Baby Banana & Kiwi
www.happyfamilybrands.com
Ingredients: organic banana, organic kiwi, ascorbic acid (vitamin C), organic lemon juice concentrate

Notes: 14g Sugar

Jennies Pound Cake Minis

Ingredients: whole eggs natural sugar cane, non-trans fat vegetable shortening, brown rice syrup, evaporated cane syrup, rice flour, potato flour, tapioca flour, glycerin, dehydrated apple powder, baking powder, pure vanilla extract, guar gum, xanthan gum, salt
Notes: DF, GF, WF, YF, 10g Sugar Very sweet and dry

Snacks - Continued

Kim & Scotts Gluten Free Bavarian Soft Pretzels

www.kimandscotts.com

Ingredients: gluten free flour blend (tapioca flour, rice flour, potato starch, granulated sugar, xanthan gum, sea salt, sorghum flour, millet flour, quinoa flour, amaranth flour, teff flour, baking powder, guar gum), eggs, filtered water, canola oil, yeast, soda

Notes: GF, 3g Sugar Made in a facility that processes wheat and milk.

Kozy Shack Original Rice Pudding

www.kozyshack.com

Ingredients: low fat milk, rice, sugar, eggs, salt, natural flavors

Notes: GF, 16g Sugar

El Mexicano Arroz con Leche Rice Pudding

Ingredients: pasteurized whole milk, rice, sugar, corn food starch, vanilla extract, cinnamon, table salt, potassium sorbate, sodium propionate, calcium acitate

Notes: 12g Sugar

Mariani Sweetened Dried Cranberries

www.mariani.com

Ingredients: cranberries, sugar

Notes: 27g Sugar Packed on equipment that also packages milk, soy, wheat, and tree nuts. Limit to just a few.

Natural Desserts All Natural Fruit Jel Dessert Mix Orange Flavor

www.

Ingredients: evaporated cane juice, vegetable gum, adipic acid, potassium citrate, natural vegan flavor, annatto color, bata carotene

Notes: GF, Vegan, 20g Sugar

Ocean Spray Craisins

www.oceanspray.com

Ingredients: cranberries, sugar

Notes: 29g Sugar High in sugar, limit to just a few. Though Ocean Spray now has a low sugar version, it includes sucralose (splenda), so is not acceptable.

Quaker Rice Cakes - Plain

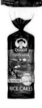

www.quakeroats.com

Ingredients: whole grain brown rice (add salt for lightly salted)

Notes: GF

Snacks - Continued

Real Foods Rice Thins
www.cornthins.com
Ingredients: wholegrain brown rice, sunflower oil, sea salt

Notes: GF, Non-GMO

Spitz Dill Pickle Sunflower Seeds
www.spitzusa.com
Ingredients: sunflower seeds, salt, sea salt, sodium diacitate, corn maltodextrin, sugar, MSG, dill weed, olive oil, citric acid, natural flavors
Notes: < 1g Sugar   The salted flavor just has sunflower seeds, salt, and olive oil, but the nice thing about the dill pickle is that it doesn't pickle your mouth.

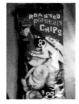

Trader Joe's Freeze Dried Banana Slices
www.traderjoes.com
Ingredients: bananas

Notes: 30g Sugar

Trader Joe's Roasted Plantain Chips
www.traderjoes.com
Ingredients: plantains, sunflower oil, salt

Notes: limit amount

Sweeteners

Ideas are included for sweeteners okay for most FMer's. Be careful to read ingredient labels, especially on Stevia, as many contain some sort of "ol" sweetener or artificial sweetener in addition to the stevia.

Florida Crystals Organic Sugar
www.floridacrystals.com
Ingredients: certified organic sugar cane

Notes: GF, Vegan, Kosher, 4g Sugar

Now Real Food Dextrose
www.nowfoods.com
Ingredients: pure Dextrose

Notes: Vegan, 4g Sugar

NuNaturals Clear Stevia
www.nunaturals.com
Ingredients: stevia extract, vegetable glycerine, 20% pure grain alcohol, water, natural flavor

Notes: SF, WF, DF, MSGF

Toothpaste/Mouthwash

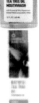

Desert Essence Tea Tree Oil Mouthwash

www.desertessence.com

Ingredients: water, glycerin (vegetable derived), polysorbte 80, maleluca alternifolia (tea tree) leaf oil, aloe barbadensis leaf juice, menthe virdis (spearmint oil) leaf oil, hamamelis virginiana (witch hazel) extract, ascorbic acid (vitamin C), calcium ascorbate, citric acid

Notes: GF, Floride-free, SLS-free Sugars N/A

Desert Essence Tea Tree Oil Toothpaste

www.desertessence.com

Ingredients: calcium carbonate, glycerin (vegetable derived), water, malaleuca alternifolia (tea tree) leaf distillate, sodium coco-sulfate, carrageenan (plant derived), gaultheria procumbens (wintergreen) leaf oil, sodium bicarbonate, Eco-Harvest malaleuca alternifolia (tea tree) leaf oil, melia azadirachta extract (neem), sea salt

Notes: GF, Floride-free, SLS-free Sugars N/A

The Honest Company Honest Toothpaste

www.honest.com

Ingredients: glycerin, calcium carbonate (mineral), water, aloe barbadensis (aloe) leaf juice, sodium lauriyl sarcosinate (coconut derived cleanser), carageenen (seaweed derived stabilizer), calcium glycerophosphate (mineral), bisabolol (botanical soother), zingiber officinale (ginger) root extract, camellia sinensis (green tea) leaf extract, ,mint flavor, sodium bicarbonate (baking soda), hydrated silica (mineral), sodium chloride (salt)

Notes: GF, Floride-free Sugars N/A

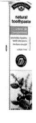

Natural Dentist Healthy Gums Antigengivitis Rinse

www.bleedinggums.com

Ingredients: aloe vera gel, purified water, vegetable glycerin, echinacea, goldenseal, calendula, citric acid, peppermint twist natural flavor, grapefruit seed extract, olivamidopropyl betaine, potassium citrate, copper chlorophyllin

Notes: Sugars N/A

Natures Gate Natural Toothpaste Crème de Mint

www.desertessence.com

Ingredients: calcium carbonate, glycerin, water, aloe barbadensis leaf juice, sodium lauroyl sarcosinate, flavor, carageenen, menthe viridi (spearmint) leaf oil, quillaja saponaria (soap bark) root extract, camellia sinensis (white tea) leaf extract, punica granatum (pomegranate) fruit extract, vaccinium macrocarpon (cranberry) fruit extract, vitis vinifera (grape seed) extract, zingiber officinial (ginger) root extract, sodium bicarbonate, hydrated silica, calcium glycerophophate, bisabolo, sodium chloride

Note: Sugars N/A

Vitamins/Supplements

Rather than list vitamins/supplements by brand, as we have done with the rest of the categories, we felt it would be easier to have them listed by supplement. We include only those which are liquid, gummy, capsule, or softgel, for absorption reasons.
Please note that we have not included sugar grams in this category.

Natrol Alpha Lipoic Acid Capsules
www.natrol.com
Inactive Ingredients: rice powder, gelatin, water, magnesium stearate

Notes:

HealthForce Nutritionals Truly Natural Vitamin C Powder
www.healthforce.com
Inactive Ingredients: areola extract, non-GMO maltodextrin as a drying agent

Notes:

Nutrition Now Vitamin C Gummy Vitamins
www.nutritionnow.com
Inactive Ingredients: glucose syrup, sucrose, gelatin, natural flavor, citric acid, color (annatto extract), lactic acid, fractionated coconut oil, beeswax

Notes: GF, DF, PF, SF

Qunol Mega CoQ10 Softgels
www.qunol.com
Inactive Ingredients: medium chain triglycerides, polysorbate 80, gelatin, glycerin, ascorbyl palmitate, purified water, annatto suspension in sunflower oil

Notes:

Biotics Research Corporation Bio-D-Mulsion Forte Liquid
www.bioticsresearch.com
Inactive Ingredients: water, gum Arabic emulsifier base, sesame oil

Notes:

Carlson Super Daily D-3 Drops
www.
Inactive Ingredients: vitamin D, vitamin E, medium chain triglyceride oil (coconut and palm source)

Notes: GF, WF, SF, CF

Vitamins/Supplements - Continued

Jarrow Vitamin D3
www.jarrow.org
Inactive Ingredients: extra virgin olive oil, gelatin, glycerin, water

Notes: GF, WF, SF, DF, EF, PF, TNF

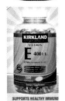

Nature Made E Softgels
www.naturemade.com
Inactive Ingredients: dl-alpha tocopheryl acetate, gelatin, glycerin, water

Notes:

Kirkland Signature E Softgels
www.costco.com
Inactive Ingredients: dl-alpha tocopheryl acetate, gelatin, glycerin, water

Notes:

Nature Made Fish Oil Softgels
www.naturemade.com
Inactive Ingredients: gelatin, glycerin, water, tocopherol

Notes:

Life Extension Low-Dose Vitamin K2 Softgels
www.lef.org
Inactive Ingredients: gelatin, medium chain triglycerides, glycerin, purified water, beeswax, carob

Notes:

Frusano Frutobalax
www.frusano.com
Ingredients: calciumcarbonate, zink glukonate, gelatin, separating agent magnesiumstearate, folic acid

Notes: GF, LF

Lil Critters Gummyvites Multivitamin
www.nnpvitamins.com
Inactive Ingredients: glucose syrup, sucrose, water, gelatin, less than 2% of: citric acid, colors (annatto extract, purple carrot juice concentrate, turmeric), fractionated coconut oil, (contains bees wax/carnauba wax), lactic acid, natural flavors
Notes: Contains tree nuts.

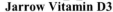

Vitamins/Supplements - Continued

Nutrition Now Multi Vites

www.nutritionnow.com

Inactive Ingredients: glucose syrup, sucrose, gelatin, natural flavors, colors (carrot and blueberry juices), annatto extract, fractionated coconut oil, beeswax

Notes: GF, WF, DF, EF, PF, SF

TwinLab Daily One Caps Multivitamin

www.twinlab.com

Inactive Ingredients: gelatin, alginic acid , crosamellose sodium, potassium, citrate, soy lecithin, medium chain triglycerides, magnesium silicate, vegetable stearic acid, silica, magnesium state, potassium aspartate

Notes:

Life Extension N-Acetyl-L-Cysteine Capsules

www.lef.org

Inactive Ingredients: gelatin, vegetable stearate, silica

Notes:

Phillips' Colon Health Probiotic

www.phillipsrelief.com

Inactive Ingredients: potato starch, gelatin, silicon dioxide

Notes:

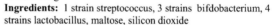

VSL #3 Probiotic

www.lef.org

Ingredients: 1 strain streptococcus, 3 strains bifdobacterium, 4 strains lactobacillus, maltose, silicon dioxide

Notes: Available at Costco or Walgreens over the pharmacy counter without a prescription.

Wraps/Pizza Crust

Double Happiness Extra Thin Rice Paper

Ingredients: rice, tapioca, salt, water

Notes:

Erawan Rice Paper (Spring Roll Wrappers)

Ingredients: rice flour, water, salt

Notes:

French Meadow Bakery Gluten-Free Tortillas

www.frenchmeadowcom

Ingredients: rice flour, tapioca starch, filtered water, glycerine, contains less than 2% of the following: corn starch, expeller pressed canola oil, salt, sugar, leavening (sodium acid pyrophosphate, baking soda, monocalcium phosphate), organic guar gum, xanthan gum

Notes: GF, 1g Sugar Manufactured on shared equipment with egg and soy.

Three Ladies Brand Rice Paper

Ingredients: rice flour, tapioca starch, water, salt

Notes: 1g Sugar

Maria & Ricardo's Gluten-Free Tortillas

www.mariaandricardos.com

Ingredients: tapioca flour, sorghum flour, potato flour, sunflower oil, leavening agents, gums, sugar, natural preservatives (per company e--mail)

Notes: GF, WF, YF, DF, Non-GMO, Vegan

Paleo Wraps

www.julianbakery.com

Inactive Ingredients: coconut meat, coconut water

Notes: GF, YF, SF, DF, Non-GMO, Vegan, 3g Sugar, BPA-Free bags

Rudi's Gluten Free Pizza Crust

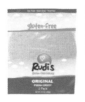

www.rudisbakery.com

Ingredients: water, rice flour, corn starch, tapioca dextrin, eggs, sugar, salt, xanthan gum, baking powder, guar gum, canola oil, rice extract

Notes: GF, SF, DF, NF

Yogurt

Chobani Greek Yogurt - Plain - Vanilla - Lemon

WWW.chobani.com
Ingredients: nonfat yogurt (cultured pasteurized nonfat milk, live and active cultures: s. thermophilus, l. bugaricvus, l. acidophilus, bifidus and l. casei), evaporated cane juice, vanilla extract, locust bean gum, pectin ,

Notes: Kosher, 4-15g Sugar

Fage Yogurt Plain

www.fage.usa
Ingredients: grade A pasteurized milk and cream, live active yogurt cultures (l. bulgaricus, s. thermophilus, l. acidophilus, bifidus, l. casei)

Notes: 7g Sugar

Mountain High Yoghurt Plain

www.mountainhighyoghurt
Ingredients: cultured pasteurized lowfat milk, pectin, contains live, active & probiotic culture3s (l. bulgaricus, s thermophilus, l. acidophilus, b. bifidus, l. casei

Notes: 16g Sugar

Stonyfield Organic Yogurt - Plain - Vanilla

www.stonyfield.com
Ingredients: cultured pasteurized organic nonfat milk, organic sugar, organic natural vanilla flavor, pectin, vitamin D3, live active cultures-l. bulgaricus, l. acidophilus, bifidus, l. casei, l. rhamnosus

Notes: 15-29g Sugar

Tillamook Yogurt - Plain - Vanilla

www.tillamook.com
Ingredients: cultured pasteurized grade A reduced fat milk, vanilla bean base (sugar, water, modified corn starch, natural flavors, citric acid, vanilla beans) sugar, modified corn starch, kosher gelatin, active yogurt cultures - l. bulgaricus, s. thermophilus, l. acidophilus, bifidus,
Notes: 30-37g Sugar

Trader Joe's Organic Greek Style NonFat Yogurt Plain

www.traderjoes.com
Ingredients: cultured pasteurized organic nonfat milk, active yogurt cultures - l. bulgaricus, s. thermophilus, l. acidophilus, l casei
Notes: 11g Sugar

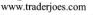

Made in the USA
Middletown, DE
23 February 2020